HEALTH21

*The health for all policy framework
for the WHO European Region*

WHO Library Cataloguing in Publication Data

Health21: the health for all policy framework for the WHO European Region

(European Health for All Series ; No. 6)

1.Health for all 2.Health policy 3.Health priorities 4.Regional health planning 5.Europe I.Series

ISBN 92 890 1349 4   (NLM Classification: WA 540 GA1)
ISSN 1012-7356

The World Health Organization is a specialized agency of the United Nations with primary responsibility for international health matters and public health. Through this Organization, which was created in 1948, the health professions of over 190 countries exchange their knowledge and experience with the aim of making possible the attainment by all citizens of the world of a level of health that will permit them to lead a socially and economically productive life.

The WHO Regional Office for Europe is one of six regional offices throughout the world, each with its own programme geared to the particular health problems of the countries it serves. The European Region embraces some 870 million people living in an area stretching from Greenland in the north and the Mediterranean in the south to the Pacific shores of the Russian Federation. The European programme of WHO therefore concentrates both on the problems associated with industrial and post-industrial society and on those faced by the emerging democracies of central and eastern Europe and the former USSR. In its strategy for attaining the goal of health for all the Regional Office is arranging its activities in three main areas: lifestyles conducive to health, a healthy environment, and appropriate services for prevention, treatment and care.

The European Region is characterized by the large number of languages spoken by its peoples, and the resulting difficulties in disseminating information to all who may need it. Applications for rights of translation of Regional Office books are therefore most welcome.

European Health for All Series No. 6

HEALTH21

The health for all policy framework for the WHO European Region

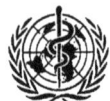

**World Health Organization
Regional Office for Europe
Copenhagen**

ISBN 92 890 1349 4
ISSN 1012-7356

The Regional Office for Europe of the World Health Organization welcomes requests for permission to reproduce or translate its publications, in part or in full. Applications and enquiries should be addressed to the Office of Publications, WHO Regional Office for Europe, Scherfigsvej 8, DK-2100 Copenhagen Ø, Denmark, which will be glad to provide the latest information on any changes made to the text, plans for new editions, and reprints and translations already available.

© **World Health Organization 1999**

Publications of the World Health Organization enjoy copyright protection in accordance with the provisions of Protocol 2 of the Universal Copyright Convention. All rights reserved.

The designations employed and the presentation of the material in this publication do not imply the expression of any opinion whatsoever on the part of the Secretariat of the World Health Organization concerning the legal status of any country, territory, city or area or of its authorities, or concerning the delimitation of its frontiers or boundaries. The names of countries or areas used in this publication are those that obtained at the time the original language edition of the book was prepared.

The mention of specific companies or of certain manufacturers' products does not imply that they are endorsed or recommended by the World Health Organization in preference to others of a similar nature that are not mentioned. Errors and omissions excepted, the names of proprietary products are distinguished by initial capital letters.

PRINTED IN DENMARK

WORLD HEALTH DECLARATION

Adopted by the world health community at the Fifty-first World Health Assembly, May 1998

I

We, the Member States of the World Health Organization (WHO), reaffirm our commitment to the principle enunciated in its Constitution that the enjoyment of the highest attainable standard of health is one of the fundamental rights of every human being; in doing so, we affirm the dignity and worth of every person, and the equal rights, equal duties and shared responsibilities of all for health.

II

We recognize that the improvement of the health and well-being of people is the ultimate aim of social and economic development. We are committed to the ethical concepts of equity, solidarity and social justice and to the incorporation of a gender perspective into our strategies. We emphasize the importance of reducing social and economic inequities in improving the health of the whole population. Therefore, it is imperative to pay the greatest attention to those most in need, burdened by ill-health, receiving inadequate services for health or affected by poverty. We reaffirm our will to promote health by addressing the basic determinants and prerequisites for health. We acknowledge that changes in the world health situation require that we give effect to the "Health-for-All Policy for the twenty-first century" **through relevant regional and national policies and strategies.**[1]

III

We recommit ourselves to strengthening, adapting and reforming, as appropriate, our health systems, including essential public health functions and services, in order to ensure universal access to health services that are based on scientific evidence, of good quality and within affordable limits, and that are sustainable for the future. We intend to ensure the availability of the essentials of primary health care as defined in the Declaration of Alma-Ata[2] and developed in the new policy. We will continue to develop health systems to respond to the current and anticipated health conditions, socioeconomic circumstances and needs of the people, communities and countries concerned, through appropriately managed public and private actions and investments for health.

---

[1] Text not highlighted in original.
[2] Adopted at the International Conference on Primary Health Care, Alma-Ata, 6–12 September 1978, and endorsed by the Thirty-second World Health Assembly in resolution WHA32.30 (May 1979).

IV

We recognize that in working towards health for all, all nations, communities, families and individuals are interdependent. As a community of nations, we will act together to meet common threats to health and to promote universal well-being.

V

We, the Member States of the World Health Organization, hereby resolve to promote and support the rights and principles, action and responsibilities enunciated in this Declaration through concerted action, full participation and partnership, calling on all peoples and institutions to share the vision of health for all in the twenty-first century, and to endeavour in common to realize it.

ACKNOWLEDGEMENTS

The new health for all policy framework for the WHO European Region is the result of a very extensive two-year process, during which drafts of this document were reviewed and input received from Member States, WHO networks and forums, United Nations agencies, international and integrational organizations, nongovernmental organizations and individual public and private sector experts. I take this opportunity to thank all those who – in many different ways and in many different capacities – contributed to the process and to the final product.

J.E. Asvall
WHO Regional Director for Europe

NOTE FOR THE READER

Chapter 1 The HFA vision outlines the vision, aims and key values of the policy for health for all (HFA) and sets out the major orientation of the renewed policy.

Chapter 2 Ensuring equity in health through solidarity in action focuses on fostering strong solidarity in health development between Member States and greater equity in health among groups within each country.

Chapters 3 and 4 set out the desired health outcome for the peoples of the Region. Chapter 3 *Better health for the 870 million people of the European Region* focuses on how to enable people to attain a higher level of health sustained over life; and Chapter 4 *Preventing and controlling disease and injury* suggests strategies to reduce the incidence, prevalence and impact of specific diseases and other causes of ill health.

Chapters 5 and 6 identify the range of strategies and actions to reach the overall goal of HFA. Chapter 5 *Multisectoral strategies for creating sustainable health* focuses on generating action from many sectors to ensure more health-promoting physical, economic, social and cultural environments for people; and Chapter 6 *An outcome-oriented health sector* on orienting the health sector to promote better health gain, equity and cost–effectiveness.

Chapter 7 Policies and mechanisms for managing change proposes ways of mobilizing political, professional and public support for HFA at all levels. It aims to create a broad societal movement for health through innovative partnerships, unifying policies, and a health development process that is tailored to the new realities of the European Region.

Chapter 8 HEALTH21 – a new opportunity for action contains the concluding comments and looks to the challenge ahead.

CONTENTS

Page

World Health Declaration v
Acknowledgements vii
Note for the reader.. viii

Chapter 1   The HFA vision 1
   1.1   The European Region of WHO at an important cross-roads in time 1
   1.2   The health for all policy and its targets.. 3
   1.3   The role of the international community in general and of WHO in particular........ 5
   1.4   Conclusion 6

Chapter 2   Ensuring equity in health through solidarity in action 7
   2.1   Achieving solidarity for health among countries in Europe 7
   2.2   Closing the health gaps within countries 13
       2.2.1   The poor.. 13
       2.2.2   The unemployed... 14
       2.2.3   Gender inequity in health 15
       2.2.4   Ethnic minorities, migrants and refugees.. 15
       2.2.5   The disabled 15

Chapter 3   Better health for the 870 million people of the European Region 19
   3.1   Life transitions and health.. 19
   3.2   Healthy start in life 21
   3.3   Health of young people 26
   3.4   Health of adult people.. 30
   3.5   Healthy aging... 33
   3.6   Dying in dignity 37

Chapter 4   Preventing and controlling disease and injury 39
   4.1   The overall burden of ill health.. 39
   4.2   Mental health 40
   4.3   Communicable diseases 43
       4.3.1   Diseases targeted for global eradication or elimination in the
              European Region... 49
       4.3.2   Control of communicable diseases through immunization 50
       4.3.3   Control of other communicable diseases 52

	4.4	Noncommunicable diseases	54
	4.5	Injury from violence and accidents	61
	4.6	Disasters	63
Chapter 5		Multisectoral strategies for creating sustainable health	67
	5.1	The biological basis of health	68
	5.2	Physical and socioeconomic determinants of health	72
		5.2.1 Physical environment	72
		5.2.2 Social and economic determinants of health	78
	5.3	Healthy lifestyles	83
		5.3.1 Healthy choices and behaviour	83
		5.3.2 Reducing harm from alcohol, drugs, and tobacco	89
	5.4	Settings to promote health	97
	5.5	Multisectoral responsibility for health	104
		5.5.1 Achieving accountability	105
		5.5.2 Action for health by other sectors	106
Chapter 6		An outcome-oriented health sector	115
	6.1	Introduction	115
	6.2	Integrating primary health care and hospital services	117
		6.2.1 Functions of integrated health services	119
		6.2.2 Organization of integrated health services	121
		6.2.3 Primary health care facilities	124
		6.2.4 Hospitals	124
	6.3	Managing for quality in health outcomes	125
		6.3.1 Application of management tools to obtain outcomes	130
		6.3.2 Planning inputs for outcomes	130
	6.4	Funding and allocation of resources for health services and care	131
		6.4.1 Financial resources	131
		6.4.2 Human resources	135
		6.4.3 Pharmaceuticals	140
		6.4.4 Medical equipment	143
	6.5	Public health infrastructure	143
		6.5.1 Public health managers	144
		6.5.2 Other public health workers	145

Chapter 7	Policies and mechanisms for managing change	147
7.1	Introduction	147
7.2	Strengthening the knowledge base for health	148
	7.2.1 Research	148
	7.2.2 Health information support	149
7.3	Mobilizing partners for health	153
	7.3.1 Governments	156
	7.3.2 Politicians	156
	7.3.3 Professionals	157
	7.3.4 Nongovernmental organizations	158
	7.3.5 Private sector	158
	7.3.6 Individual citizens	159
	7.3.7 Bringing partners together for action	159
7.4	Planning, implementing and evaluating HFA policies	162
	7.4.1 Providing a clear map of the way forward	164
	7.4.2 Creating awareness	164
	7.4.3 Agreeing on the process	164
	7.4.4 Searching for consensus	165
	7.4.5 Setting targets	165
	7.4.6 Achieving transparency	166
	7.4.7 Legitimizing the process	166
	7.4.8 Creating new alliances	167
	7.4.9 Broadening the range of instruments for policy implementation	167
	7.4.10 Coordinating, monitoring and evaluating progress	168
Chapter 8	HEALTH21 – a new opportunity for action	169
Annex 1	Relationship between global and regional HFA targets	173
Annex 2	21 targets for the 21st century and suggested areas for formulating indicators	177
Annex 3	Schedule of main events 1998–2005	203
Annex 4	List of abbreviations	207
Annex 5	Glossary of terms	209
Annex 6	Bibliography	219

Chapter 1

The HFA vision

1.1 The European Region of WHO at an important crossroads in time

Some eight hundred and seventy million people live within the European Region of the World Health Organization (WHO), in 51 countries covering an area from Greenland in the west to the Pacific coast of the Russian Federation in the east. Like the rest of the world, the Region is undergoing profound change, and the recent rapid development of information and other technologies may well cause a new "industrial revolution" with profound consequences, the full extent of which cannot be foreseen.

The Region is one of great contrasts. While all its Member States are committed to the principles of democracy, human rights and political pluralism, it contains both some highly developed and rich countries and some poor or very poor ones. Many are still struggling with the consequences of the democratic, social and economic transition that began in the early 1990s.

Over the past decade the number of Member States in the Region has increased from 31 to 51, and the extent and scope of its problems have grown. Persistent problems of poverty and unemployment are exacerbating inequities and in many countries are giving rise to deteriorating lifestyles, increasing violence and weakened social cohesion. Doubts about the quality of health and other services, and an imbalance between the demand for and the availability of resources, have in many countries caused fears that hard-won social safety nets and benefits may be dismantled. Increasing globalization, decentralization and pluralism, while offering new opportunities, have often given the impression that individuals, and even governments, have less and less control over the decisions which affect health.

During the 1990s, the average life expectancy of the 870 million people in the European Region actually declined for the first time since the Second World War, largely owing to a deterioration in health status in the newly independent states (NIS) and some countries of central and eastern Europe (CCEE). In almost all countries, there has been an increase in the health gap between more and less advantaged socioeconomic groups. While the situation varies from country to country, noncommunicable and communicable diseases, accidents, mental health problems and complications related to pregnancy and child birth are the major health problems in the Region; their relative priority differs according to the parameter (mortality, disability, etc.) used for the assessment. Too many people are dying prematurely, when the knowledge and means of avoiding this are available.

In considering the future health of Europe, it is also important to recognize areas of uncertainty. Most significant in this respect are phenomena such as migration and social conflict. Information technology, genetics, biotechnology and microtechnology are rapidly developing and will affect the way we communicate, the way we work, our environment and the way health services are delivered.

However, there is also cause for much hope and optimism. Although not all tensions have disappeared, the many wars seen in the Region during the first half of the 1990s have been curbed. Thus the twenty-first century could well become the first where countries are able to make human development their main priority. People and countries are starting to come to terms with the initial trauma of the recent changes, and stronger civic societies are emerging. Solid infrastructures for transport and communications, and for the provision of public amenities such as water and electricity, housing and other services, are already in place throughout most of the Region.

Furthermore, the Region has a well educated population. Its information base, research capacity and know-how are among the best in the world, and the current huge expansion of communication technology will allow this knowledge to be quickly disseminated. Scientific and technological advances are already showing the way to new and improved tools for health gain. The expansion of the European Union (EU) offers new opportunities for collaboration and mutual support between countries.

Most importantly, the European Region of WHO now has almost 15 years of experience in together designing, implementing, monitoring and evaluating a joint outcome-focused, targeted and innovative policy in health that integrates efforts to promote healthy lifestyles, a healthy environment, and quality-oriented and cost-effective health care. Ample practical experience in European countries has demonstrated the strong advantage of this approach, and a vast body of knowledge has been built up about how best to organize ways of making policies for health for all (HFA). An intensive development effort has changed "health promotion" from being a vague idea to become a major approach to improve the population's health. This comprises an umbrella of "healthy public policy" and a series of concrete, detailed strategies and methods to promote mental health, healthy nutrition and physical activity, as well as to reduce the health risks related to tobacco, alcohol and drug use. The Frankfurt (1989) and Helsinki (1994) conferences have created a Region-wide strategy to promote a healthy environment, and this has been actively followed up by virtually every Member State through multisectoral national environment and health action plans (NEHAPs).

A health outcome-based approach to clinical medicine, entailing continuous monitoring of selected quality criteria and feedback to users through appropriate information systems, has been developed.

This has revealed a formidable potential for improving the quality of patient care, increasing the cost–benefit of health services, and, ultimately, releasing resources that can be used to introduce new health care technologies. Other health care reform experiments have pointed to better ways of organizing and financing health care. Last but not least, a new strategy has been developed, turning the idea of HFA into a broad social movement through the creation of collaborative networks. These act as vehicles to mobilize many sectors and organizations to work together in permanently organized partnerships of regions, cities, schools, worksites, health institutions and professionals, nongovernmental organizations (NGOs), etc., that join forces to make the HFA idea a reality in their individual areas of work.

In this situation, the Member States have a strong obligation to take action to halt and reverse the deteriorating trends in health by grasping the new opportunities that this collective experience has created. Only by working together can this scenario of "hope and optimism" become reality.

1.2 The health for all policy and its targets

The policy for "Health for all in the twenty-first century", adopted by the world community in May 1998, aims to realize the vision of health for all – a vision born in the World Health Assembly in 1977 and launched at the Alma-Ata Conference in 1978. It sets out, for the first two decades of the twenty-first century, global priorities and ten targets that will create the conditions for people worldwide to reach and maintain the highest attainable level of health throughout their lives.

The regional policy for HFA is a response to the World Health Declaration's call for regional and national policies to be developed on the basis of the global policy (see inside cover page) and is in line with the regional HFA plan of action (i.e. schedule of main events) adopted in 1991, which asked for a renewed policy to be presented to the WHO Regional Committee for Europe in 1998. The World Health Declaration itself calls on all Member States to take action nationally and internationally.

This HFA policy document provides the framework for taking up the challenges of achieving better health by applying the best strategies that have emerged from the Region's collective experience during the past 10–15 years. The arguments contained within this new policy for the European Region demonstrate the essential relationship between health, poverty and social cohesion and show how health and health development efforts are now emerging as important factors in contributing to greater social cohesion between and within the populations of the Region.

The HEALTH21 policy for the European Region of WHO has the following main elements:

The **one constant goal** is to achieve full health potential for all.[3]

---

[3] See Glossary of terms (Annex 5) for WHO definitions of health and health potential.

Two main aims for better health guide efforts towards this ultimate goal:

- promoting and protecting people's health throughout the course of their lives;
- reducing the incidence of and suffering from the main diseases and injuries.

Three basic values form the ethical foundation:

- health as a fundamental human right;
- equity in health and solidarity in action between countries, between groups of people within countries and between genders; and
- participation by and accountability of individuals, groups and communities and of institutions, organizations and sectors in health development.

Four main strategies for action have been chosen to ensure that scientific, economic, social and political sustainability drive the implementation of HEALTH21:

- multisectoral strategies to tackle the determinants of health, taking into account physical, economic, social, cultural, and gender perspectives and ensuring the use of health impact assessments;
- health-outcome-driven programmes and investments for health development and clinical care;
- integrated family- and community-oriented primary health care, supported by a flexible and responsive hospital system; and
- a participatory health development process that involves relevant partners for health, at all levels – home, school and worksite, local community and country – and that promotes joint decision-making, implementation and accountability.

Twenty-one HFA targets have been set for the European Region. They will provide the benchmarks against which to measure progress in improving and protecting health and in reducing health risks. The 21 HFA targets together constitute the framework for developing health policies in the European Region. They are not meant to be a prescriptive list, but together they make up the essence of the European policy. These targets meet the challenge of the World Health Declaration and reflect those set out in the global policy for "Health for all in the twenty-first century". However, they specifically address the situation and needs within the European Region, as well as the regional response to them. Annex 1 depicts the relationship between the global and regional targets. Where the European targets have been quantified, their values express the average for the whole Region or, in some cases (where specified) for subgroups of countries (see Annex 2).

Countries, subnational entities, cities and local communities, etc. in the European Region are expected to adapt these targets to meet their own local conditions, needs and capacities.

1.3 The role of the international community in general and of WHO in particular

The European Region of WHO has a formidable resource in the many organizations that can work with countries to support their efforts. The European Union (EU), an integrational organization with a strong mandate for multisectoral action for health, has a large potential for contributing to this development. The Council of Europe, with its essential concern for democracy, human rights and ethics, can be a major force in ensuring that basic ethical values are indeed defended in international agreements guiding individual countries and local communities. The World Bank, the European Bank for Reconstruction and Development (EBRD) and other funding institutions, including donor agencies in many European countries, can provide essential support for financing major new investments in line with the policy and the different needs of individual countries. The organizations of the United Nations family, through their support to national policy formulation and concrete assistance with programmes and projects in many of the countries of the Region, can help to bring cohesion and clear direction to international and national efforts in line with the policy. The vast number of NGOs, both at the regional level and within countries, can find inspiration and guidance for their work through the policy and greatly enhance the effectiveness of their efforts by joining international, national or local partnerships based on the principles of HFA.

Through its Constitution, WHO has a special mandate to promote closer cooperation for health development, both internationally and in its work with individual countries. Needless to say, this task has to take into account the realities of the European Region at the end of the twentieth century and the need to establish cooperation with different partners that respects their specific mandates and is based on mutual trust and a spirit of partnership.

On this basis, the Regional Office for Europe will work closely with WHO headquarters and other regional offices, as well as with its international partners, so that European Member States can derive maximum benefit from the wider experience and potential for action inherent in the global nature of WHO. Against this background, there will be five major roles for WHO's Regional Office for Europe to play in support of implementation of the policy in countries:

1. act as a "health conscience", defending the principle of health as a basic human right, identifying and drawing attention to persistent or emerging concerns related to people's health;
2. function as a major centre for information on health and health development;
3. promote the HFA policy throughout the Region and ensure its periodic updating;
4. provide up-to-date evidence-based tools that countries can use to turn HFA-oriented policies into action; and
5. work as a catalyst for action by:

- providing technical cooperation with Member States – this can be strengthened through the establishment of a strong "WHO function" in every country, to ensure the mutually beneficial exchange of experience between the country and the regional health organization;

- exercising leadership in Region-wide efforts to eradicate, eliminate or control diseases that are major threats to public health, such as epidemics of communicable diseases and pandemics such as tobacco-related diseases;

- promoting HFA-oriented action with many partners through networks across the European Region;

- facilitating the coordination of emergency preparedness for and response to public health disasters in the Region.

1.4 Conclusion

As we stand on the brink of the twenty-first century, we have a strong obligation to take action to improve the health of the 870 million people of the Region. HEALTH21 provides the framework for accepting that challenge by applying the best strategies that have emerged from Europe's collective experience during the past 10–15 years.

It is not a vision beyond our grasp – it can be done! Experience has shown that countries with vastly differing political, social, economic and cultural conditions can develop and implement HFA policies designed to put health high on the agenda – and when they do, they stand to gain from a fundamental change for the better. The major challenge for the 51 Member States in the Region is now to use the new regional HFA policy as an inspirational guide to update, as necessary, their own policies and targets.

Throughout the Region, many local communities have shown great initiative and imagination in using the HFA ideas to mobilize people to promote and protect their health. Excellent examples can be seen of the public and private sectors exploring the possibilities for health gain. Thousands of health professionals and many of their organizations have introduced innovative approaches to improving the quality of care and working more closely with other disciplines to find new ways of meeting the challenges. The dynamic and rapidly expanding "Healthy Cities" movement, in particular, has demonstrated a formidable potential for systematic, sustainable and innovative mobilization of local communities in every Member State.

Clearly focused and committed action is now needed to transform the vision of HFA into a practical and sustainable reality in every one of the 51 Member States in the Region. The experience, the know-how and many of the tools for influencing the determinants of health are all there; what is needed now is strong leadership and the political will to pick them up and use them.

Chapter 2

Ensuring equity in health through solidarity in action

> Target 1 – Solidarity for health in the European Region
> Target 2 – Equity in health

Policy-making is agreeing on a vision for the future, how to get there and how to use resources and mobilize partners appropriately. The choice between various policy options must, however, be made on the basis of a clear set of values, and these must be rooted in the strong ethical foundation of the Universal Declaration of Human Rights. As mentioned in Chapter 1, equity in health and solidarity in action are two such key ethical values in the HFA policy. In the European Region they appear in two dimensions, both of which require a strong programmatic response. One dimension is the large and growing inequity between Member States, the other is the wide – and now often widening – gap in health among groups within each country.

2.1 Achieving solidarity for health among countries in Europe

As already mentioned, the WHO European Region includes some of the richest countries in the world and others which are extremely poor; even worse, a much larger group of countries now belong to the less well-to-do than ten years ago. In 1996, per capita gross national product (GNP) ranged from US $340 to over US $45 000, and the further east one goes, the bleaker the situation is (Fig. 1).

According to the *Human development report 1997*, issued by the United Nations Development Programme (UNDP), "Eastern Europe and the countries of the Commonwealth of Independent

States (CIS) in economic transition have seen the greatest deterioration in the past decade. Income poverty has spread from a small part of their population to about a third – 120 million people live below a poverty line of US $4 a day."

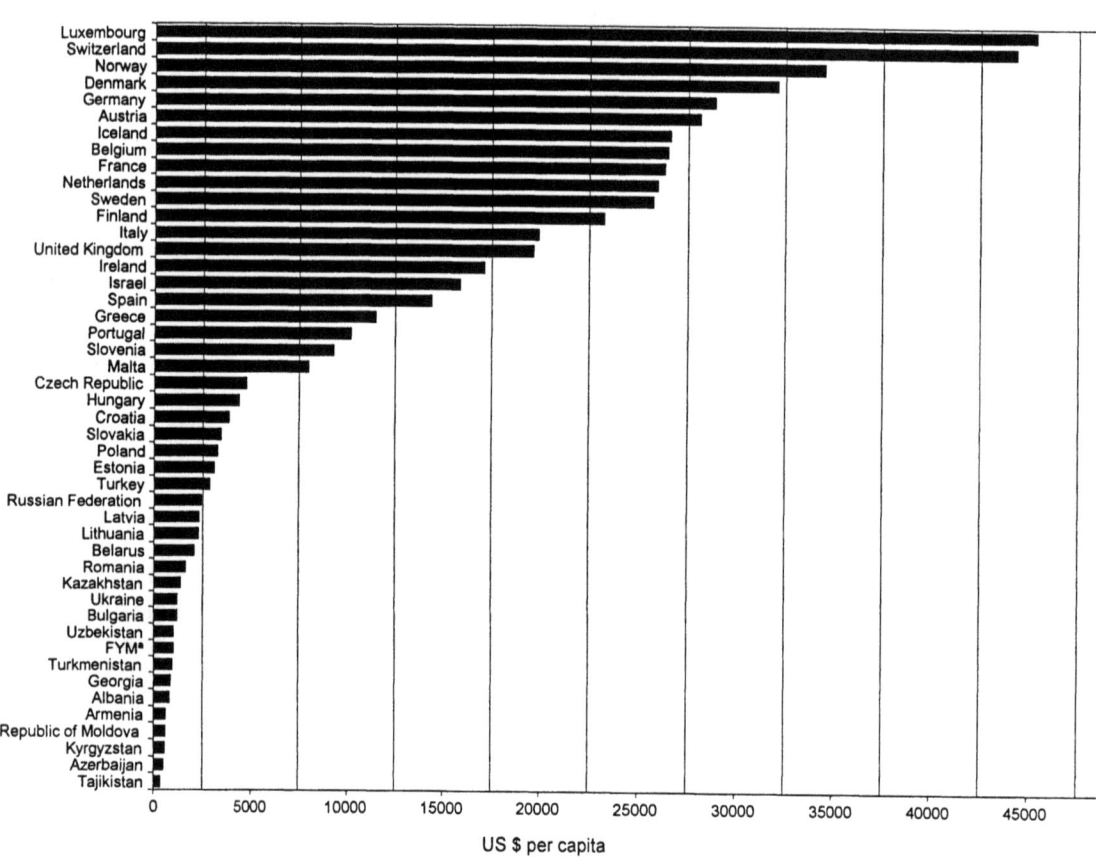

Fig. 1. Per capita GNP, 1996[4]

a The Former Yugoslav Republic of Macedonia.

The economic upheavals and the wars in the CCEE and NIS during the 1990s have increased the gap in health status between countries in the Region, as reflected in the wide range of variations in many health indicators (Fig. 2). Today, for example, average lifespan varies by 15.3 years between Iceland, at 79.3 years, and Turkmenistan, at 64 years.

---

[4] Most country data are from the latest World Bank Atlas and refer to 1996. For Malta data refer to the latest available year (1993); for Azerbaijan a 1997 estimate is given. Bosnia and Herzegovina and San Marino were excluded as the latest data were from 1991 (the pre-war period) and 1983, respectively.

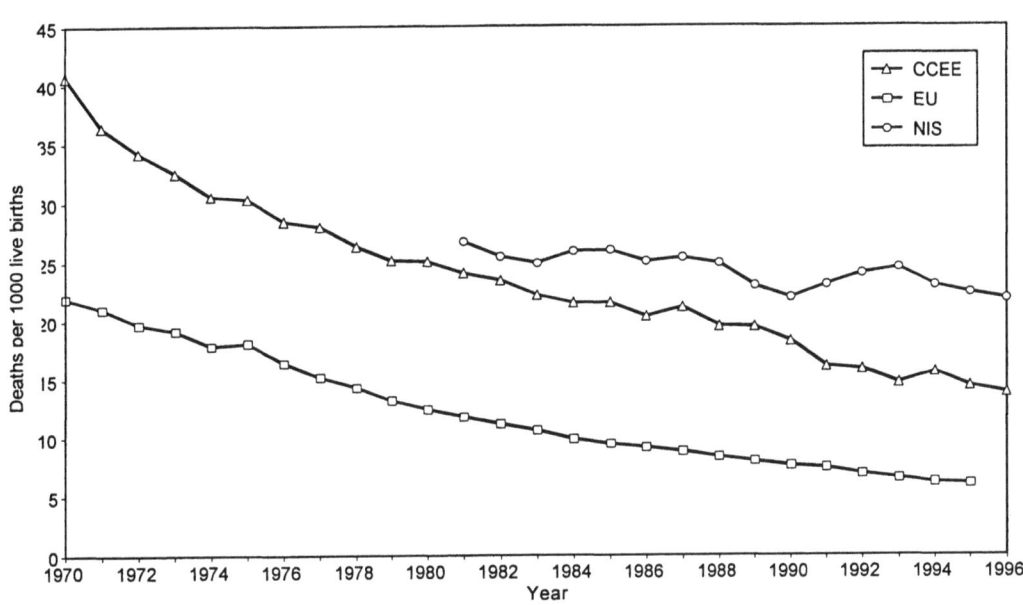

Fig. 2. Infant mortality in subregional groups of countries in the European Region 1970–1996

In the context of the 1998 World Health Declaration, and its commitment to the highest attainable level of HFA, it is difficult to see such differentials in economic and health experience, closely linked as they are, in anything other than human rights terms. The Member States in the European Region of WHO are part of the global family of nations, and the persistence and even growth of variations in health status and the quality of life enjoyed by different members of that family, on this scale, is unacceptable and requires much stronger emphasis to be placed on the promotion of equity in health in the twenty-first century.

Furthermore, the massive and rapid movement of people across national borders in today's Europe is increasing manyfold the potential for the spread of communicable diseases. The growing influence of a powerful entertainment industry and of other technological and cultural factors on the behavioural and environmental determinants for health make joint, concerted action a must for countries of the Region. A Region-wide movement for health that uses a common policy which includes a strong component of helping the worst-off countries to catch up with the best is, ultimately, in the self-interest of every Member State.

Although increased external assistance has been provided to the CCEE and NIS during the 1990s, the total amount of external assistance in the health field has been far lower than needed, and the total impact has often been disappointingly low. At times the degree of excellence of individual experts sent to help has not matched that of those whom they were supposed to assist. Much more could certainly have been done, for example, about dealing with the debts some governments have inherited. With some notable exceptions, the donor countries, international organizations and funding agencies that have provided external assistance have often worked too much in isolation – either at their own wish or at that of the recipient country's government. Not only has this created additional burdens on scarce planning resources in receiving countries, it has also carried the considerable risk that priority-setting might be more influenced by donor interests than by a carefully worked out development plan. However, there have also been good examples of sound, well coordinated health development plans based on a national HFA policy and elaborated in close partnership between the government, international partners and donor agencies (e.g. the MANAS programme, described below).

MANAS: KYRGYZSTAN'S COMPREHENSIVE HEALTH CARE REFORM PROGRAMME

After first formulating a national HFA policy, Kyrgyzstan developed a comprehensive reform programme in 1994–1996 through a participatory process involving all stakeholders in the country. The programme represents an example of outcome-oriented, integrated health sector development. It is designed to improve health gain. To strengthen primary care, various polyclinics for different population groups have been merged, with family physicians replacing specialists at that level. Secondary care is being rationalized by reducing the number of beds and merging or closing down some facilities. Substitution policies are being used in some areas, such as introducing short-term chemotherapy for tuberculosis to reduce the number of hospital beds required.

The state budget continues to be the main source of funding, in order to maintain as much equity as possible. The method of allocating funds has been shifted from a norm-based system towards the use of a needs-based formula. Payment mechanisms are changing towards more incentive-based arrangements, such as capitation payments for primary care providers and global budgets for inpatient care, with the introduction of more autonomy. In future, it is planned to use contracts with a purchaser/provider split, although the Government is moving forward with caution until the necessary regulatory mechanisms are in place.

Medical and nursing education are undergoing reforms, and a programme is being implemented to retrain existing specialists so that they can work as family physicians. Information systems are being upgraded to meet the new requirements.

Source: MANAS – National programme on health care reforms. Bishkek, Ministry of Health of Kyrgyzstan, 1996.

Major disasters create emergencies – natural, man-made or complex – that often require rapid and large-scale outside help to the affected country or countries. During the 1990s, the European Region has experienced armed conflicts in ten Member States, all of them inflicting huge suffering and damage to the physical and mental health of the affected populations. Responding to this situation, hundreds of organizations and many donor countries have been involved in emergency assistance, often in a very uncoordinated way. However, there have also been positive signs of more willingness to cooperate and skills in doing so, and evidence that new tools are being developed to speed up and facilitate needs assessment and the provision of emergency aid.

> **TARGET 1 – SOLIDARITY FOR HEALTH IN THE EUROPEAN REGION**
>
> BY THE YEAR 2020, THE PRESENT GAP IN HEALTH STATUS BETWEEN MEMBER STATES OF THE EUROPEAN REGION SHOULD BE REDUCED BY AT LEAST ONE THIRD.
>
> In particular:
>
> 1.1 the gap in life expectancy between the third of European countries with the highest and the third of countries with the lowest life expectancy levels should be reduced by at least 30%;
>
> 1.2 the range of values for major indicators of morbidity, disability and mortality among groups of countries should be reduced through accelerated improvement of the situation in those that are disadvantaged.

PROPOSED STRATEGIES

If inequities are to be lessened and the security and cohesion of Europe maintained, a much stronger collective effort must be made by Member States, integrational, governmental and NGOs to increase the volume, effectiveness and coordination of support to countries most in need in the Region.

Countries and organizations providing assistance need to work much more together towards common goals. The quality and appropriateness of the technical experts sent to receiving countries should be carefully monitored by providers, and experts should be selected on the basis of clear evidence of a high degree of excellence in their home country. Donors have a responsibility to ensure that the practices they advocate for receiving countries would be acceptable in their own country, particularly in relation to industrial development. Industry itself – both individual companies and industry groups/associations – has similarly a strong moral responsibility to observe and promote the same principle.

More formal partnership agreements between the major integrational and intergovernmental organizations and funding agencies would be an important step forward, and these should be followed up through concrete collaborative frameworks for each receiving country. Such partnerships promote a more integrated approach to capacity-building, policy development and resource mobilization for health. All national donor agencies, investment banks, integrational and international organizations that contribute to health development in the European Region should aim towards setting a common development agenda. A good example of practical cooperation on shared priorities is the European Environment and Health Committee (EEHC). The possibility of establishing "consortia" of donor countries and organizations to develop common approaches and pool resources should be considered; the Interagency Immunization Coordinating Committee (IICC), and the recently established Task Force on the Human Immunodeficiency Virus and Sexually Transmitted Diseases, are good examples of this. The EU now has a stronger mandate for public health and its membership is expanding, which should facilitate closer collaboration between a considerable number of countries.

Both donors and receiving countries should aim at achieving the goals of the "20/20 initiative", which advocates that 20% of overall development assistance should be allocated to social sector activities, and that receiving countries should allocate, on average, 20% of their national budgets (net of aid) to basic social services.[5] The Human Development Index, based on life expectancy, educational attainment and income, provides a useful guide for prioritizing support to countries most in need.

Receiving countries, for their part, should give very high priority to the formulation of HFA policies and, on that basis, make health and development plans for the medium and long terms through which all external support from countries, agencies and organizations can be managed in a closely coordinated way and directed towards issues of priority concern.

For every country, true solidarity and enlightened self-interest lie in sharing a common health policy and common values. The concept of HFA provides such a framework, and every country must be able to contribute to and profit from HFA and the technical work of WHO at global and regional levels. Therefore, in order to make HFA better known and to strengthen countries' individual links to the Regional Office, each country ought to consider establishing "a WHO country function". This could be a unit within the ministry of health, a collaborating centre, or a national expert group which would be responsible for systematically assessing the relevance and possible follow-up of new policies and scientific advice emanating from WHO, and for bringing that information to the attention of top decision-makers in government. This function would also include a systematic review of all new developments in public health and clinical medicine in their country that would be of interest to WHO, so that it could spread such knowledge to other countries.

The process should not stop there: in order to mobilize public support for such efforts, countries should encourage a wider public debate about health and socioeconomic inequities and their implications in terms of human suffering and injustice, diminished solidarity and social cohesion, and sustainable economic growth in the Region. Such a debate should lead to a better understanding of the human, social, economic and cultural benefits of closing the gaps and raising the overall level of health, as well as to the mobilization of resources and technical expertise to reduce the current inequities. Much of the basic information needed to hold this discussion is available, as a result of ongoing monitoring of progress towards HFA by WHO and of work done by organizations such as the World Bank, UNDP, United Nations Children's Fund (UNICEF), the EU, and NGOs. It is particularly important that this debate involves all organizations and individuals with an interest in health. In particular, ministries of foreign affairs, who are

---

[5] *The 20/20 Initiative. Achieving universal access to basic social services for sustainable human development.* New York, UNICEF, 1994.

responsible for decisions regarding foreign support, need to place the reduction of inequities higher on their agenda. In the private sector, multinational corporations (including their shareholders, consumers of their products and the multinational mass media) need to be made aware of the possible impact of their policies on health status in disadvantaged countries and populations.

Tools, mechanisms, and structures to support and enforce such policies include the capacity for policy analysis, structures for cooperation, and methods for health impact assessment. The latter methodology should be scientifically sound but kept as simple as possible, so that it can be effectively implemented on a wide scale.

The health of people affected by emergencies can be improved if countries are better prepared for them and if assistance given during the humanitarian and transitional phases is focused more clearly on the longer term. In the post-emergency phase, health action can be used as an effective entry point to promote solidarity and social cohesion, and it can play a significant role in promoting post-conflict dialogue and reconciliation.

2.2 Closing the health gaps within countries

2.2.1 The poor

Poverty – whether defined by income, socioeconomic status, living conditions or educational level – is the largest single determinant of ill health. Living in poverty is correlated with higher rates of substance use (tobacco, alcohol and illegal drugs), depression, suicide, antisocial behaviour and violence, an increased risk of food insecurity and a wide range of physical complaints. Large – and in fact increasing – numbers of people in European societies today are at risk of experiencing poverty sometime in their lives.

Even in affluent societies, health inequalities increase with widening socioeconomic disparities, in a social gradient running across all socioeconomic groups, the whole society and throughout life. Thus, although national health policy should give top priority to those who are worst off, it should also address the unequal distribution among all social groups of the benefits accruing from socioeconomic growth and from a more fair distribution of societal goods (e.g. access to education, employment).

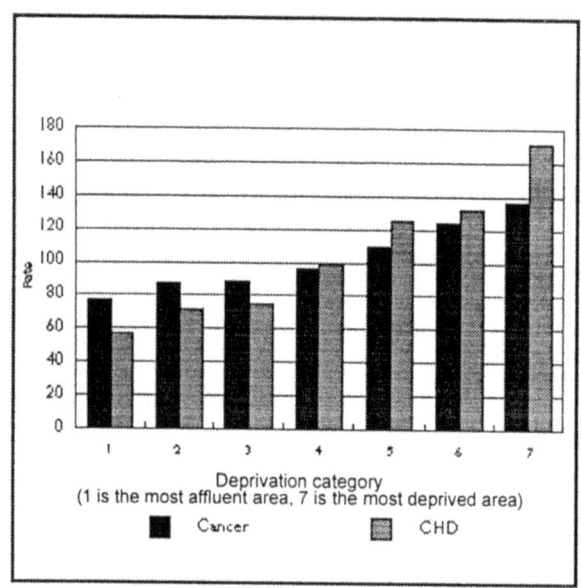

Fig. 3. Standardized mortality rates for cancer and coronary heart disease among people under 65 by area of deprivation, 1991

Source: Common Services Agency, Information and Statistics Division.

2.2.2 The unemployed

Among employed people, there is a clear association between the grade of employment, on the one hand, and mortality and morbidity (including rates of absence due to sickness), on the other. This relationship remains when adjustment is made for factors such as level of education and tenure of housing. It seems to be explained by the higher levels of work control, demands and support enjoyed in higher grades.

Both unemployment and work insecurity have detrimental effects on health, increasing the risk of psychological and physical disorders and suicide. In the younger age groups, work insecurity is associated with poor health, irrespective of any relationship between social class and unemployment. Both the long-term steady rise of unemployment in most countries of western Europe, and its sudden steep rise in NIS, are a cause of grave concern for equity in health.

Education is an important determinant of health. Educational levels produce a gradient in mortality and morbidity similar to that produced by income. The material and cultural resources of a family have a major influence on a child's educational attainment. There is thus a strong social class gradient in educational qualifications – and this, in turn, is a strong predictor of subsequent occupation and income. Children who attain higher levels of education or technical training have much better chances in health, as well as in occupation and income.

2.2.3 Gender inequity in health

Gender issues should be considered in conjunction with those of differences in socioeconomic groups. Women live longer than men (on average 5–7 years more in western Europe and about 7–15 years in eastern countries). Their double burden of work at home and in the workplace, however, takes a heavy toll in terms of morbidity, and they are more likely than men to suffer from depression and anxiety. Gender-specific issues such as maternal deaths are of grave concern in a number of Member States. On the other hand, men are more prone to accidents, for example, and it is the health of working-age men that has deteriorated most in CCEE/NIS in recent years. Rape and wife battering, although grossly under-reported, show alarming proportions in the large majority of countries; in fact, in industrialized countries domestic assaults have been reported to cause more injury to women than traffic accidents, rape and muggings combined. Section 3.4 deals with gender issues and related strategies in more detail.

2.2.4 Ethnic minorities, migrants and refugees

Special groups including ethnic minorities, gypsies, migrants and refugees are at particular risk of poor health status. Their needs often receive far less attention, and they cannot always be reached through usual health and welfare channels. This problem is increasing in many countries.

2.2.5 The disabled

Physically or mentally disabled people are also a group with very special problems and needs. This subject is dealt with in detail in section 5.4.

The HFA monitoring exercise shows that countries now report not only on geographic differences but also on variations according to occupation and level of education. Some refer to the effects of unemployment and issues such as nutrition and housing. Countries affected by war and its aftermath, in particular, refer to the situation regarding migrants' and refugees' health. About one quarter of the Members States report that they have been improving their information systems to reflect inequities in health, and some have been developing new indicators for the purpose. There has also been a considerable increase in research on the issue, but this relates mainly to the measurement of inequities: there is comparatively little research on the effectiveness of interventions to close the gaps.

> **TARGET 2 – EQUITY IN HEALTH**
>
> BY THE YEAR 2020, THE HEALTH GAP BETWEEN SOCIOECONOMIC GROUPS WITHIN COUNTRIES SHOULD BE REDUCED BY AT LEAST ONE FOURTH IN ALL MEMBER STATES, BY SUBSTANTIALLY IMPROVING THE LEVEL OF HEALTH OF DISADVANTAGED GROUPS.
>
> In particular:
>
> 2.1 the gap in life expectancy between socioeconomic groups should be reduced by at least 25%;
>
> 2.2 the values for major indicators of morbidity, disability and mortality in groups across the socioeconomic gradient should be more equitably distributed;
>
> 2.3 socioeconomic conditions that produce adverse health effects, notably differences in income, educational achievement and access to the labour market, should be substantially improved;
>
> 2.4 the proportion of the population living in poverty should be greatly reduced;
>
> 2.5 people having special needs as a result of their health, social or economic circumstances should be protected from exclusion and given easy access to appropriate care.

PROPOSED STRATEGIES

One very important strategy for dealing with inequities in health is the systematic, broad effort (referred to above) to build public support for more enlightened socioeconomic policies which address the basic inequalities in income and social goods (e.g. access to free health care, education, etc.).

A prerequisite for addressing the whole issue in a serious way is to be able to correctly assess the health divide and its causes; special efforts should therefore be made to identify groups at particular risk of poor health and premature death, and to analyse the causes of social differences in health. Existing sources of information could often be better used, but many countries need to modify their health information systems in order to record socioeconomic variables more precisely and to include more health information in existing socioeconomic statistics. Much more attention needs to be paid to monitoring and evaluating the effectiveness of interventions to close the health gaps.

> **ASSESSMENT OF THE HEALTH DIVIDE AND ITS CAUSES**
>
> 1. As part of the Global Initiative for Equity in Health and Health Care, launched by WHO and the Swedish International Development Agency (SIDA), Lithuania (for example) has identified more than 20 existing sources of health and/or socioeconomic indicators which can be used to map inequities in that country.
>
> 2. Finland, the Netherlands, Spain, Sweden and the United Kingdom have all recently set up special commissions to assess the health divide.
>
> 3. Norway is trying to develop new indicators to better reflect inequities in health, and Sweden stresses the need for an integrated approach to gender and socioeconomic indicators.
>
> 4. An ambitious effort has been initiated in the Netherlands to report on and forecast public health status, in order to inform the policy-making process.
>
> Source: *Exploring the process of health policy development in Europe*. Copenhagen, WHO Regional Office for Europe (in press).

Determinants of health

A heightened level of commitment and more forceful action is needed to deal with the determinants of health. The policies that are most successful in sustaining and improving the health of the population are those which deal with economic growth, human development and health in an integrated way. Income differentials, health choices and environmental protection are all variables that are amenable to public policy and where changes can lead to improved health and wellbeing for the whole population. Fiscal and legal measures are powerful regulatory instruments for tackling the underlying causes of ill health. Chapter 5 considers in more detail strategies to influence the physical, environmental and socioeconomic determinants of health, notably income distribution, employment and education.

If such regulations are to be implemented effectively, they must be upheld by all the sectors and institutions concerned and they must, above all, enjoy public support and confidence. This can be achieved by mobilizing society at large and generating informed discussion through effective communication. Public policy needs to be assessed for its impact on health equity.

Selecting a starting point

There are several possible starting points for formulating plans to tackle inequities in health. Each country will select that which is most appropriate to its situation. One way is to focus on specific health problems where significant differences between socioeconomic groups have been observed. This has the advantage of being easily understood by the public and health professionals. A second approach is based on recent evidence which shows that tackling the risk factors and underlying causes of inequities in health is more appropriate when wide income differences are apparent, or when there are pockets of severe unemployment or poor housing, particularly at the local level. A third approach is to start by identifying groups at particular risk. There is evidence that risk factors accumulate in the same social groups, and this approach enables several risk factors to be addressed at the same time. In overall health policies, differential targets may be set for these groups.

In most cases, a mix of approaches will be adopted. Countries can also consider building an equity element into all major ongoing programmes, although this might not always be a sufficiently focused approach.

For groups at particular risk, health policies should be culturally and gender-sensitive, ensuring access to appropriate care and support.

Outreach services

The provision of outreach services and the reduction of financial and other barriers to service access can improve the health of people living in poverty (these are discussed in more detail in Chapter 6). Outreach services are particularly important for reaching vulnerable groups such as the elderly, ethnic minorities, etc. who may not be aware of how to access the support they need or may be hindered from using such services by social, psychological, or even physical barriers. Breaking the cycle of poverty through early intervention in the lives of infants and children can lead to substantial health gains for present and future generations (this is discussed in more detail in Chapter 4).

Integrated policies are needed to support vulnerable groups. The health of migrants and refugees can be improved if access is ensured to a system of family health services, adequate housing, and educational and employment opportunities. As far as possible, vulnerable groups must be guaranteed financial coverage which secures their rights to health care at the same level as the rest of the population. Integrated programmes developed at community level – involving a broad range of sectors and agencies – can be effective in tailoring services to the specific cultural, attitudinal and other characteristics of the groups concerned.

The health of people affected by emergencies can be improved if humanitarian assistance is both speedy and effective, and if national and international policies exist which cut down unnecessary bureaucracy and provide for an immediate flow of funds and the support of experts and relief workers. The role of the health sector is to provide the evidence that such policies are necessary, to help develop partnerships with the relevant sectors and to support them in the evaluation of their policies.

Chapter 3

Better health for the 870 million people of the European Region

> Target 3 – Healthy start in life
> Target 4 – Health of young people
> Target 5 – Healthy aging

HFA aims to give all people the opportunity of a high quality of life throughout their life. People's welfare is related to the degree to which their health permits them to participate in, and benefit from, life and development. Functional health and quality of life go hand in hand throughout life. The focus of this chapter is on ensuring better health outcomes for the population.

3.1 Life transitions and health

Life contains a series of critical transitions which are marked by particular life events (see box). Some life events and circumstances are specific to women or concern them predominantly, such as child bearing, multiple paid and unpaid roles, and the menopause.

Adopting a life course approach to developing policies for health recognizes the complex interactions between such life events, biological risks, and health determinants. The way these elements interact has implications for people's health from the moment they are born to when they die. Health can be depleted at any stage over the course of life through chance, circumstance and choice. A life course approach is more effective in reaching all groups of the population than only developing policies and programmes to deal with each health problem as they occur (this tends to be a more fragmented way of working and can lead to unnecessary duplication, over-specialization of services for some population groups, and under-attention to others). A life course approach ensures better health outcomes for the entire population in the medium and longer terms.

> **CRITICAL PERIODS IN HUMAN DEVELOPMENT:**
> - birth
> - transition from primary to secondary school
> - school examinations
> - leaving parental home
> - establishing own residence
> - entry to labour market
> - transition to parenthood
> - job insecurity, change, or loss
> - onset of chronic illness
> - exit from labour market
> - loss of spouse and close friends
>
> *Source*: Bartley, M. et al. Socioeconomic determinants of health. Health and the life course: why safety nets matter. *British medical journal*, **314**: 1194 (1997) (first and last items added).

At each transition point in the course of life, supportive action at both the macro and micro levels can enhance health and wellbeing. Some actions are common to the health and wellbeing of all groups, and at the macro level social, economic and other public policies need to create environments which ensure that people at all times of life are better able to reach their full health potential. On a micro level, action initiated in particular settings e.g. the home, school, and workplace, can be very effective (see Chapter 5). Health and social services, and in particular primary health care (PHC) services focused on reaching out to families in their homes, to workers at their workplaces, and to local community groups with special needs, are important entry points for systematically supporting individuals and communities over the lifespan, and in particular during critical periods (this is dealt with in more detail in Chapter 6).

Investing early in health protection typically pays off later. Important aspects of physical and mental health are developed early in life, with a legacy from the mother in relation to prenatal development; from both parents in regard to genetic endowment and postnatal care; and from the quality of the social and physical environments in the early years of life. Therefore, health and welfare policies must have a sharp focus and broad vision on the early years of life.

Children's chances of a healthy life are unequal throughout the European Region. Parental poverty, in particular, can start a chain of social risk that damages health over the entire life course, and investing in the socioeconomic wellbeing of parents and families is therefore crucial to the promotion of health and development. Throughout life, welfare policies need to provide not only safety nets but also springboards to offset earlier disadvantage.

Over the entire life course, societal assets contributing to better health are: economic stability; social cohesion; the development of coping skills and opportunities for people to influence their environment; and a decrease in frustration and failure. Most serious adult diseases have long courses of development; the health effects of environmental hazards and health-damaging lifestyles often do not manifest themselves until some considerable time after people have been exposed to them, usually in adult or older age. For many people and groups, the interplay of multiple disadvantages, individual choice and life circumstances results in an increased likelihood of premature death and disability.

The remainder of this chapter deals with four specific age groups. Three targets have been set in relation to a healthy start in life (including reproductive health), children and youth, and older people, as they are stages within the life course which offer considerable opportunity for protecting, promoting and maintaining health.

In addition to the life events experienced by all or most people, specific events occurring to some people at various points in their lifespan may result in disability. A brief analysis of the situation in the Region is given and some proposals put forward for strategies to realize health opportunities for people with disabilities (see section 5.4 for settings and opportunities for disabled people). The chapter concludes with a short discussion on how people's right to die in dignity can be protected.

3.2   Healthy start in life

Giving children a healthy start in life must be a top priority for any society. This subchapter focuses on creating health for infants and young children up to school age. It includes life events such as birth; physical development; learning to walk and speak; acquiring basic social and health values; discovering the environment; and strengthening bonds to parents and people close to the family.

The chances of a child being born healthy are unequal throughout the Region, and this is also true of the chances of a child surviving its first year of life. Most western European countries have, at national level over the past fifteen years, met the regional HFA target of reduced infant mortality, but even in the richest countries there are significant inequalities between social groups. The high infant mortality rates in some countries in the eastern part of the Region give rise to particular concern. An unwelcome pregnancy is a risk factor, and the considerable number of teenage pregnancies, for instance, is an important problem in many countries. Abortion is still used as a major means of contraception in some countries – a practice that is unacceptable at the turn of the century. Maternal mortality remains a considerable problem in many Member States.

A healthy birth establishes the basis for a healthy life, and pre- and perinatal services may contribute significantly to helping mothers and infants cope with this crucial life event. Pregnancy and delivery are natural physiological processes – although at times they go wrong – and should be regarded as such by health professionals. The better a mother's state of education, health and nutrition, and the higher her socioeconomic living standard and the quality of health-related services she receives, the greater is the chance of a successful pregnancy. A healthy start in life is related to the lifestyles and parenthood skills of both parents. Post-partum depression can affect not only the mother but also the father and can be a factor in violence in the family.

> **THE EUROPEAN TASK FORCE FOR PERINATAL CARE**, initiated in Venice in 1998, reinforced the importance of basic values and principles in the European context. Care for normal pregnancy and birth should be: de-medicalized; based on the use of evidence-based appropriate technology; regionalized; multidisciplinary, holistic, family-centred and culturally appropriate; and involve women in decision-making. While these values and principles are being promoted throughout the European Region, Belarus and the Republic of Moldova stand out as leaders in the field and have included many of the principles in their national perinatal care policies.
>
> Source: *Workshop on perinatal care: report on a WHO expert meeting, Venice, Italy, 16–18 April 1998.* Copenhagen, WHO Regional Office for Europe, 1998 (document EUR/ICP/FMLY 01 02 02).

There is considerable inequity in the provision and quality of perinatal and postnatal services in the Region. Whereas some countries spend large amounts of money on increasing the life expectancy of very low birth-weight infants, the basic requirement of ensuring a healthy birth is not met in large parts of the Region. The very success of perinatal medicine in ensuring survival at ever lower birth weights has been associated with a greater number of children being born with special needs, raising important ethical questions.

Birth weight, which is related to income (but also to other factors, such as smoking), is a marker for indices of deprivation and represents accumulated risk over generations. Even when compared with others in the same social class, a child's reduced birth weight is associated with a greater risk of physical ill health, including death from coronary heart disease (CHD) and psychological ill health in adult life. Birth weight is also related to subsequent social circumstances in childhood and up to early adulthood, including adult occupational social class. The first year of life is crucial for healthy physical and mental development and for health later in life, and children born into disadvantaged home and family circumstances are at higher risk of poor growth and development.

The bonds to parents and people close to the family should be strengthened. Parents and other close people have an important role to play in conveying basic health and social values to children of this age group. In times of crisis or difficulty, or situations where there may only be one parent, parents and those taking care of children do not always have the necessary parenting skills or support. Europe faces important changes in family structures. The number of "traditional families" is decreasing, as a result of higher rates of family breakdowns and increases in the proportion of births to unmarried mothers. Divorce rates have risen markedly in CCEE, with especially significant increases in Belarus, Estonia, the Republic of Moldova, the Russian Federation and Slovakia. Children can suffer if families split up. The pressures are greater on families in some parts of western Europe, where traditional social support networks are deteriorating, than in southern and eastern parts of the Region, where they are still strong.

Infant and child abuse has lasting and traumatic effects on the individual's mental health. The number of marginalized street children is increasing in the Region, and the problem does not always receive as much attention as it should. Children from immigrant families, refugee families, families staying illegally in foreign countries and homeless families are most at risk of becoming street children and hence of delinquency, prostitution, truancy, drug use, poverty, violence and begging.

TARGET 3 – HEALTHY START IN LIFE

BY THE YEAR 2020, ALL NEWBORN BABIES, INFANTS AND PRE-SCHOOL CHILDREN IN THE REGION SHOULD HAVE BETTER HEALTH, ENSURING A HEALTHY START IN LIFE.

In particular:

3.1 all Member States should ensure improvements in access to appropriate reproductive health, antenatal, perinatal and child health services;

3.2 the infant mortality rate should not exceed 20 per 1000 live births in any country; countries with rates currently below 20 per 1000 should strive to reach 10 or below;

3.3 countries with rates currently below 10 per 1000 should increase the proportion of newborn babies free from congenital disease or disability;

3.4 mortality and disability from accidents and violence in under 5-year-olds should be reduced by at least 50%;

3.5 the proportion of children born weighing less than 2500 g should be reduced by at least 20%, and the differences between countries should be significantly reduced.

PROPOSED STRATEGIES

The question of how to deal with the underlying social and economic determinants, in order to decrease infant mortality within and among Member States, is discussed in Chapter 5. To ensure that pregnancies are wanted and carried through in the best possible condition, it is important to have a good family planning programme for the population (including genetic counselling, when appropriate). For pregnant women, essential services include basic medical check-ups and good help for parents-to-be with stopping smoking, guidance on nutrition, and psychological and physical advice on pregnancy, delivery and child care.

One proven strategy for improving women's and infant health is the application of the Safe Motherhood Initiative.

> **THE SAFE MOTHERHOOD INITIATIVE** was launched in 1987 by the international health community, including WHO, UNICEF, the United Nations Population Fund, the World Bank and many local and international NGOs around the world, in order to reduce maternal and infant mortality and morbidity. In particular, it aims to: ensure skilled attendance at delivery; improve access to maternal health services; improve the quality of maternal health services; prevent unwanted pregnancy; address unsafe abortion; and measure progress through effective data collection systems. Since 1995 the CARAK project has been promoting the Initiative in two pilot districts in each of the central Asian republics and in Azerbaijan; this has already resulted in a drop in infections, haemorrhages and abortions, and an increase in the use of contraceptives.
>
> Source: *Maternal Health and Safe Motherhood Programme: progress report 1993–1995*. Geneva, World Health Organization, 1995 (document WHO/FRH/MSM/96.14).

A healthy birth should be assisted by well trained midwives, with back-up services from obstetricians only in case of need. Pre- and perinatal care should rely on evidence-based essential technologies only, with more sophisticated technology reserved for special, clearly identified needs; potential iatrogenic side effects should always be kept in mind. The obstetrical quality of perinatal care can be greatly improved through the use of appropriate indicators and monitoring, including the use of telematics. Separating mothers and infants at birth, and putting too much emphasis on regularity, discipline and hygiene, all interfere with protective physiological mechanisms and should therefore be avoided; in this context, the WHO criteria for baby-friendly hospitals (see below) are a useful source of advice. Attention must be paid to the lifestyles and the psychosocial wellbeing of both parents. Future mothers, fathers and other family members should refrain from smoking, and the mother should avoid the use of drugs and alcohol. Good and timely immunization coverage is a basic disease prevention mechanism and should always be ensured (details can be found in Chapter 4).

Breastfeeding provides optimal nutrition, creates strong bonds between mothers and children, reinforces the immune system and gives additional protection against infectious diseases and allergies during childhood. Almost every mother has the capacity to produce milk which exactly meets all the nutritional requirements of her particular baby for about six months. This is true even under the conditions generating severe and long-lasting physiological and psychological stress which are currently found in many countries in the Region.

A safe, stable and supportive home environment is of particular importance for infants and young children, since they spend a lot of time in and near the home and are particularly vulnerable to the health hazards found there: communicable diseases; water-, food- and animal-borne infections; diseases caused by poor sanitary conditions; chemical hazards from air, water, and soil pollution; and physical hazards in the home, neighbourhood and traffic. Creating an environment which allows children to develop their physical, emotional and social potential is an investment with long-term health effects. This environment should be smoke-free, since passive smoking has a clear detrimental effect on children's health. Social policies should give support to families in need, allowing them to create a nurturing, stable and safe home environment.

> **THE BABY-FRIENDLY HOSPITAL INITIATIVE (BFHI)** was launched by WHO and UNICEF in 1991 at a meeting of the International Paediatric Association in Ankara, with the following objectives:
>
> - to enable mothers to make an informed choice about how to feed their newborn babies;
> - to support early initiation of breastfeeding;
> - to promote exclusive breastfeeding for the first six months;
> - to ensure cessation of the free and low-cost supply of infant formula to hospitals;
> - to include, possibly at a later stage and where needed, other mother and infant health care issues.
>
> This global network aims to give every baby the best start in life by creating a health care environment where breastfeeding is the norm, thus helping to reduce the levels of infant morbidity and mortality in each country.
>
> In the European Region of WHO, as at September 1998, there were 314 baby-friendly hospitals in 24 countries but the aim is to include all hospitals in the Region.

A family health nurse making home visits can be highly instrumental in helping parents create a healthy, psychosocially stimulating and active environment for the infant, as well as one which prevents injuries at home.

The private sector can contribute to health, for example by manufacturing healthy toys which enhance children's imagination and development.

In the first seven years of life, stable social relationships are known to contribute significantly to a person's psychological make-up and the ability to cope with stressful events throughout life. The experience of profound and loving human relationships builds a strong health resource for the whole life course. Parenting education for mothers and fathers could be part of health services. Establishing partner and family counselling, as well as school education programmes in group dynamics and conflict solving, may have positive health effects in the case of parents separating.

The kindergarten and similar child care facilities are excellent settings in which to convey basic health values and develop social skills, and where equity, solidarity and human dignity, for example, can be experienced and taught. Such facilities can also contribute to the healthy development of young children by providing a model of a healthy physical and social environment; by encouraging children to prepare healthy food together; by teaching them "life skills" of social interaction; and by supporting and introducing basic hygienic behaviour. Countries need to make much greater efforts to ensure that all such institutions have systematic programmes to meet these requirements, including staff trained for the purpose.

Supporting vulnerable and at-risk children, especially those who may not already be within the social welfare system, requires effective community and outreach services. Working together with other partners, including the social sector, children's welfare services, NGOs and charities can make for more effective action. A very important, but difficult task is to develop programmes in all Member States to prevent infant and child abuse, and to rehabilitate children who have suffered abuse. This requires a new openness in many societies to talk about problems which hitherto have been "swept under the carpet".

WHO/UNICEF GUIDELINES ON INTEGRATED MANAGEMENT OF CHILDHOOD ILLNESS

The guidelines aim to reduce mortality and the frequency and severity of illness and disability in countries, and to contribute to better growth and development. The interventions focus on the quality of the care provided by outpatient health facilities and at community level.

The initiative is considered to have the potential to make a large impact on the global burden of disease and to be extremely cost-effective. It is based on three components:

- improving the case management practices of health staff, by providing guidelines on the integrated management of childhood illness adapted to the local context and by organizing activities to promote their use;
- improving the health infrastructure required for effective management of childhood illness, including the supply and management of essential drugs and vaccines and supervisory capabilities at national and district levels;
- improving family and community practices.

3.3 Health of young people

The following section deals with the health potentials arising during childhood and adolescence, or the period from entering school to entering the job market. It also takes account of life events such as acquiring social and health skills, puberty, and taking up responsibilities in society.

Entering school changes the everyday life of many children. Childhood and adolescence are stages of life during which there are particular periods of intellectual and physical development and during which lifelong social and health skills are acquired. The ability of young people to make decisions about their health behaviour is greatest when they can participate in influencing their own social, physical and educational environment.

Young people's psychological wellbeing, and consequently their health, is closely linked to the quality of their relationships with family members, other adults and peers. A caring and supportive family, accepting and understanding friends, and other significant adults with whom young people can interact are crucial for healthy development and a positive self-image. High self-esteem and good problem-solving abilities, including those of resolving conflict, are valuable resources for coping throughout life.

The physical and emotional changes experienced by young people during puberty give rise to new feelings and perceptions. Such changes occur at differing speeds and with varying intensity, depending on the individual. During this period feelings and attitudes can be experienced at a more intense level. There is a strong drive to conform to the norms of the peer group. Many experiences are very positive and should be seen as a natural part of maturation.

Young people may also be highly vulnerable to particular risks, however, such as drug-taking and tobacco and alcohol use, or behaviour related to sexual maturation (see section 5.3). Unprotected sexual activity is still leading to many unwanted pregnancies, abortions and sexually transmitted diseases (STDs), including HIV infection. In many parts of the Region factual, unbiased sex education is not provided either in schools or in other settings, placing young people in vulnerable situations during a period of life when experimental activity is normal. Unnecessary emotional stress is created by the lack of information and understanding about issues to do with sexuality, bodily changes and functions, and emotional feelings. Inadequate provision of confidential health services for young people can also inhibit them from accessing appropriate health care and advice.

Decreased physical activity and unhealthy eating habits have led to an increase in obesity among young people in many countries which, if continued into adulthood (as is often the case), poses a substantial risk to health.

Unfortunately, violent behaviour is now becoming more frequent in the lives of many young people and adolescents. Injuries, both intentional (self-inflicted and as a result of intentional violence) and unintentional, are currently the leading cause of death in children above one year of age and in adolescents. Rates are higher in males than females. More and more children in the Region are subjected to sexual exploitation and sexual abuse. At the World Congress against Commercial Sexual Exploitation of Children (Stockholm, August 1996), Member States committed themselves to concerted action at the local, national, regional and international levels to bring an end to the sexual exploitation of children.

The growth of the telecommunications, media and information industry means that young people throughout the world are being exposed to similar products, messages, and values. Advertising, media and music are not just forms of entertainment, they also act as vehicles for marketing people, products, ideas and behaviour which can either promote or damage health. Much of this entertainment is counter-productive to health; for instance, there is a strong correlation between tobacco advertising and smoking levels in adolescents. Increased exposure to television, films and computer games may be associated with the increasing incidence of violence in young peoples' lives, as well as a lowering of physical activity.

> ## TARGET 4 – HEALTH OF YOUNG PEOPLE[6]
>
> BY THE YEAR 2020, YOUNG PEOPLE IN THE REGION SHOULD BE HEALTHIER AND BETTER ABLE TO FULFIL THEIR ROLES IN SOCIETY.
>
> In particular:
>
> 4.1 children and adolescents should have better life skills and the capacity to make healthy choices;
>
> 4.2 mortality and disability from violence and accidents[7] involving young people should be reduced by at least 50%;
>
> 4.3 the proportion of young people engaging in harmful forms of behaviour[8] such as drug, tobacco, and alcohol consumption should be substantially reduced;
>
> 4.4 the incidence of teenage pregnancies should be reduced by at least one third.

PROPOSED STRATEGIES

A sense of coherence and belonging

Health is created if people are confident that life is manageable and meaningful, and if they have adequate resources (mental, physical, emotional, social and material) to meet whatever demands are placed on them. As a sense of coherence and belonging must be built up from infancy and childhood, experiences in the family, kindergarten, school and health care environments have an important role to play in ensuring that young people get a consistent message and acquire the resources and coping skills that life requires.

Schools are an important setting in which health can be created and sustained. Young people's perception of health can be greatly enhanced by the content of the formal teaching curriculum. Action to protect and promote health can be brought to life in the school's physical environment. On a wider level, the school influences the perceptions, attitudes, actions and behaviour not only of pupils but also of teachers, parents, health care workers and local communities. All aspects of organizational life contribute to physical, social and emotional health; moreover, the young learn best about responsibility and empowerment through direct participation in decision-making. The European "health-promoting school" approach combines these elements, and this concept should be introduced in all schools in the 51 Member States in the Region.

---

[6] Up to 18 years of age.
[7] See also target 9, "Reducing injury from violence and accidents".
[8] See also target 12, "Reducing harm from alcohol, drugs and tobacco".

Health services

The health of older children and adolescents can be improved if health policies for young people are more comprehensive, incorporating public health, health promotion, and the integrated management of illness in children (WHO/UNICEF guidelines on integrated management of childhood illness aim to reduce mortality and the frequency and severity of illness and disability in CCEE, and to contribute to better growth and development).

Services need to be taken into the settings of daily life (the home environment, schools and other educational institutions, and recreational facilities). They should be based on the concepts of PHC and family-oriented health services. Community-based injury prevention programmes, reaching out to all settings in which children and adolescents live, should cover the whole Region.

Chronic diseases, functional disorders with physical manifestations, psychosomatic complaints and mental disorders can all be more effectively addressed if medical care is combined with psychological, social and educational services. Special prevention and intervention programmes for the young must be developed to deal with issues such as drug use, suicide, alcohol consumption and accidents, and they should be developed in partnership with social, educational, and other relevant sectors.

The health of older children and adolescents can be improved if barriers to health service access are reduced through information campaigns and by protecting young people's confidentiality, arranging for varied hours of business, organizing outreach services, etc. One particularly important channel is the family health nurse who visits people in their homes and can identify problems at an early stage and give sensible advice, both to children and to their parents.

Healthy lifestyles

Effective strategies to promote lifelong healthy eating habits can help to counteract the increase in obesity, foodborne diseases and allergies. Interventions should include growth monitoring, counselling on correct complementary feeding, fortification of foods with micronutrients, and securing regular supplies of food. Moderate physical activity and recreation can enhance young people's physical, mental and social wellbeing. Sports associations, youth clubs, etc. are important settings for health and social interaction and should be particularly supported in disadvantaged communities.

Because of young people's susceptibility to advertising, marketing and new products, industry can be an important partner for health for this age group; the health sector, however, has a responsibility to stand firmly against products which put the health of young people at risk. Strategies to combat the use of alcohol, tobacco, and illicit drugs are described in Chapter 6. Policies to regulate the media can prevent young people from being exposed to violence and risk-taking behaviour. Peer-led education has been shown to be often an effective, innovative way to empower young people to better resist harmful behaviour patterns and adopt more healthy lifestyles.

Marginalized young people

Member States have a particular responsibility to nurture an environment, attitudes and practices which are responsive to children's rights; to give high priority to action against the commercial sexual exploitation of children; and to allocate adequate resources for these purposes. In many countries, closer cooperation between all sectors of society is needed to prevent children from entering the sex trade and to strengthen the role of families in protecting children against commercial sexual exploitation. As these children are likely to have fallen outside normal health and welfare channels, special outreach and community services – including those in recreational and health care settings – are an effective locus for action.

3.4 Health of adult people

The following section deals with the health potential of adult people, from when they set out to enter the labour market up to the time when they usually leave it again. This stage of life entails some forty years and includes life events such as taking up employment; parenting; citizenship; caring for parents; witnessing children leave the house; and leaving employment.

Over the years, the nature of such life events has undergone considerable change. For many adults in Europe, economic and social conditions are unsatisfactory. An increasing number of people spend some part of their lives either under- or unemployed, due to trends such as the globalization of trade and technological development. For those who are employed, declining stable employment and the emergence of new types of work mean that large categories of workers are vulnerable to job insecurity: these include foreign workers, immigrants, ethnic minorities, older workers and women with young children. Family structures tend to be less sustainable, and many new forms of living together are being seen.

With regard to the working environment, too much emphasis is placed at present on short-term economic considerations, rather than on the longer-term human investment which creates socially productive roles for people of working age. A high level of job insecurity may create short-term economic benefits but worsens the health status of working people – and those they care for – in the long term, thus increasing the pressure on the health system.

A major barrier to the achievement of HFA is inequality, both between men and women, among women in different parts of the European Region, and among social classes and ethnic groups. Women and men are affected by many of the same conditions, but they experience them differently. Poverty and economic dependence, violence, negative attitudes and other forms of discrimination, limited power over sexual and reproductive life, and lack of influence in decision-making, are all factors which impact adversely on women's health.

Women sometimes have different and unequal access to and use of basic health services and opportunities to protect, promote and maintain their health. Health policies and programmes often perpetuate a gender stereotype and may not fully take account of women's lack of autonomy regarding their health. Complications related to pregnancy and childbirth are among the leading causes of mortality and morbidity of women of reproductive age in some countries with economies in transition. Unsafe abortions threaten the lives of a large number of women – in the more eastern part of the Region in particular – representing a grave public health problem; it is primarily the poorest and youngest who take the highest risk.

A larger proportion of the workforce than previously is now female, and the increase in working mothers and dual-worker households has implications for caring for children and older people. Traditionally women have fulfilled this role, and in many countries they continue to do so as well as working outside the home.

Poor housing and community environments (see Chapter 5) prevent many adults from adopting health-promoting behaviour. For low-income women, smoking may be a way of coping with the stress of poverty or monotonous work conditions. In poor districts, many factors make healthy lifestyles more difficult:

- there are fewer recreation areas;
- a heightened sense of crime inhibits people from going outdoors, socializing, engaging in a physical activity;
- access to public transport is poorer;
- the types of food recommended in health-promoting strategies are not available or affordable;
- primary health care services are less available than in more advantaged areas.

PROPOSED STRATEGIES

Policies for health need to help people cope with the diseases they may encounter during adult life. Preventing disease and premature death by addressing the underlying causes and risk factors should, however, be an important focus of every health strategy. A number of risk factors are common to cardiovascular diseases, cancer and diabetes (and, to some extent, chronic respiratory disease): these are smoking, alcohol use, unhealthy diet, lack of physical exercise and, increasingly, stress. Therefore, rather than concentrating preventive efforts on individual factors only, an integrated approach should be adopted to tackle all the major risk factors, within the framework of a broader health promotion and disease prevention strategy as outlined in Chapter 5.

Ensuring job security maintains and improves the health of working people. The resulting increase in individual productivity and decrease in health care costs also lead to long-term economic benefits. As outlined in Chapter 5, the health of working people can also be improved if labour market policies, while ensuring job security, promote flexible and family-friendly employment practices, giving workers the opportunity to participate in the labour market and meet personal and family responsibilities. Providing opportunities for parental leave, part-time work and job-sharing can promote the health of workers and families.

Health and wellbeing of women

By supporting and acting on the commitments in various international agreements (especially the Beijing Declaration and Platform for Action, the Programme of Action of the International Conference on Population and Development, the Copenhagen Declaration on Social Development, and the Convention on the Elimination of All Forms of Discrimination against Women), governments, in collaboration with NGOs and employers' and workers' organizations, and with the support of international institutions, can promote and protect the health of women.

Women's health can be improved through the provision of more accessible, available and affordable PHC services of high quality, including those for sexual and reproductive health (e.g. family planning information and services), with particular attention being paid to maternal and emergency obstetric care. Recognizing and dealing with the health impact of unsafe abortion, as agreed in the Programme of Action of the International Conference on Population and Development, is a major public health issue for some countries and requires, as mentioned earlier, a well planned family planning programme.

Redesigning health information services and training programmes for health workers so that they are gender-sensitive, reflect the user's perspectives with regard to interpersonal and communications skills and take into account the user's right to privacy and confidentiality, are approaches which can ensure that a greater number of women have access to good health services and are treated in a way appropriate to their needs.

To promote equality between men and women, among women in different parts of the European Region, and among women in different social classes and ethnic groups, all policies in the health sector and other fields should incorporate a gender perspective. Particular attention should be paid to developing policies and programmes that support men and women in their various roles and responsibilities – as individuals, parents, workers and carers, among others – and that remove gender-related barriers to health and human development.

A GENDER PERSPECTIVE – RECOGNIZING THE NEEDS OF WOMEN AND MEN

A gender perspective is essential to health policy because it:

- recognizes the need for the full participation of women and men in decision-making;
- gives equal weight to the knowledge, values and experiences of women and men;
- ensures that both women and men identify their health needs and priorities, and acknowledges that certain health problems are unique to, or have more serious implications, for men or women;
- leads to a better understanding of the causes of ill health;
- results in more effective interventions to improve health;
- contributes to the attainment of greater equity in health and health care.

Ensuring a safe home and community

Adequate housing is a prerequisite for health, but people's housing needs usually change over the course of their lives and housing should be adapted to meet these changing needs, including the increase in work from home. Recreation areas, safe streets, and access to public transport and basic amenities and services are essential resources for a healthy and safe community and strong social networks, and they should be maintained and improved. Health can be improved if PHC services increase the percentage of immunization coverage and focus on the early detection of cardiovascular diseases and cancer and the rehabilitation of people with chronic diseases. Services should reach out to those most in need (see Chapter 6).

Healthy lifestyles

With regard to healthy lifestyles, adults are often responsible for the care of others. The choices they make and are enabled to make with regard to healthy lifestyles can therefore influence the health of a number of people. Ensuring access to safe and affordable food, disseminating information, labelling food (in particular genetically modified foods) in an appropriate way, and providing education and training in the safe preparation of food can promote and protect the health of individuals and families. Moderate physical activity is one of the cornerstones of good health for adult people. The health benefits of physical activity are reviewed in Chapter 5. The design of daily living facilities should enhance moderate physical activity.

3.5 Healthy aging

Eighteen out of the 20 countries in the world with the highest percentages of older people are in the European Region of WHO: in those countries, between 13.2% and 17.9% of the population are over 65 years old. Within the next 20 years, there will be a highly significant increase in the proportion of people in this age group, with the fastest growing population in most countries being those who are very old (i.e. aged 80 years and above). In the next 30 years, the proportion of people aged over 80 years (as a share of the over-65 population) will increase, in Europe as a whole, from 22% to over 30%.

Aging is a natural physiological process in which the body undergoes a series of changes. There is a very wide range of variation in terms of what this means for individuals and their ability to lead an active and fulfilling life. Many older people remain active and fully independent until very close to the end of their lives. Major threats to the health of older people are dementia, depression and suicide, cancer, cardiovascular diseases, osteoporosis, incontinence and injuries.

This section challenges some of the myths surrounding aging and points out how strategies to create safer communities and more supportive health and social policies and services can help older people.

Although older people are more vulnerable to the above threats, they are by no means an inevitable part of the process of aging for everyone. In many parts of the Region, too much emphasis is placed on the decline of functions, too little on the opportunities to stay active. Little attention is paid to the health effects of declining social roles throughout the lifespan. Whereas adults have to shoulder multiple social and economic roles, they are often ill-prepared for a socially fulfilling life after regular employment comes to an end, children have moved out of the house and body functions are declining. Much ill health is created through the misconception that aging is accompanied by inactivity, and that it only starts at the age of 65.

There are many opportunities to stay active and interested in life. Education levels of people aged 65 and above are increasing, and there are new opportunities for older people to continue education. In some countries, possibly as a result of higher levels of education, older people have established political groupings and pensioner action groups to voice their demands in relation to the development of social and health policies and services. On a broad scale however, too few efforts are being made to meet the changing needs and expectations of older people, and to prepare for an increasingly aging Europe.

Women are living longer than men, but these extra years are often accompanied by chronic illness, disability and difficulties in functioning independently, especially in the age group of the "old-olds", (i.e. people aged 80 years and over). Dependence has physical, economic, psychological and social dimensions which have a powerful negative impact on the quality of life of the very old, an age group of which women currently represent some 60–64%. One reason for the gender-based difference in functional ability may be that, as muscle mass becomes less, women fall below the "critical threshold" earlier than men do.

Women tend to have fewer earnings and savings than men, a trend which is likely to continue over the next decade, with implications for public expenditure and women's health and quality of life.

The physical environment is an important determinant of older people's ability to maintain their independence, both in their homes and when going out into the local community. Housing, transport and the design of local services are at present often obstacles to maintaining the functional levels of many elderly people, and a hindrance to sustaining their social networks. In particular, many transport systems in Europe cannot readily be used by older people; access to buses and subways is often poor.

Most older citizens want to stay in their homes as long as possible. However, there is a lack of appropriate home care services in a number of countries in the Region – especially for people with dementia. In many countries, older people do not have access to preventive care services. Such services are very important for older people, however, as is illustrated by the very high demand for injury-related care. In general, rehabilitation has proved to be of great use in helping older people to lead independent lives and in increasing their autonomy and quality of life.

Older people consume a disproportionately large proportion of all prescribed drugs. In some countries, extensive drug use appears to be a substitute for the lack of rehabilitation services. Compliance in taking medicaments can be a big problem, especially for older people living on their own.

The current curricula for training health professionals are often based solely on medical treatment and hospital care; this contributes to the provision of considerable amounts of inappropriate services for older people in the Region.

TARGET 5 – HEALTHY AGING

BY THE YEAR 2020, PEOPLE OVER 65 SHOULD HAVE THE OPPORTUNITY OF ENJOYING THEIR FULL HEALTH POTENTIAL AND PLAYING AN ACTIVE SOCIAL ROLE.

In particular:

5.1 there should be an increase of at least 20% in life expectancy and in disability-free life expectancy at age 65 years;

5.2 there should be an increase of at least 50% in the proportion of people at age 80 years enjoying a level of health in a home environment that permits them to maintain autonomy, self-esteem and their place in society.

PROPOSED STRATEGIES

Healthy aging

Health can be improved if European societies take active steps to change the negative image of aging, and if people in middle age have opportunities to slowly reduce their working commitments while increasing the social roles that they could carry on after regular employment has ceased. Older people are a great resource for their families and society, and they can make a large contribution to the quality of life and wellbeing of the family. Their experience and accumulated wisdom are invaluable assets in child-rearing and to other adults in the family, benefiting society as a whole and their immediate community long after they have ceased regular employment. However, this potential is rarely being fully exploited today.

Local communities

Older people need to be facilitated to take part in community and social activities. By working together, older people, their families, carers, the local community and NGOs can find innovative ways to ensure that they continue to lead an active and interesting life. Such strategies may contribute to strengthening an older person's capacity to cope with the loss of a spouse, family members or friends. The physical environment should enable older people to participate in social networks and experience daily interaction with other people. Health can be improved if town planning and transport systems are designed with all potential users in mind, and if signposting is sufficiently large and clear to meet the needs of older people.

Health and social support

Given the demographic profile of European societies, social and other policies aimed at maintaining autonomy in old age and encouraging solidarity between the generations are becoming ever more important. Policies are also needed to ensure an adequate income and subsidies to cover the costs of basic goods such as food and fuel, particularly in some eastern parts of the Region. Effective integrated health and social policies are community-oriented, participatory, locally based and needs-led, and build on health assets. Case studies have shown that mobilizing cities and other local communities to improve health care and other services for older people is an effective strategy.

Health services

A large measure of independence can be maintained through the use of relatively low-cost devices and services. Systematic interventions to improve hearing, mobility (hip replacement), sight and chewing ability (dentures) may be of great benefit in terms of wellbeing, autonomy and activity and should receive much higher priority. The quality of life of older people and their families can be improved, while dramatically reducing expensive care for this population group, if services are gender-sensitive and based on PHC; and if they reach out actively to every older person in the local community (e.g. through a family health nurse, see Chapter 6). Key service elements include an assessment of both the health needs and assets of each older person and his or her environment. If the older person wishes to stay at home, support should be given to adapt the home to his or her needs; home help should assist the older person in maintaining his or her autonomy. This should also be the prime goal of nursing homes. Good coordination of health and social services in the community ensures continuity of care, supports people in their home environment as long as possible, and means that care institutions are used only when necessary.

Training curricula in PHC need to take much more account of the needs and assets of older people and be oriented towards the main goal of maintaining their autonomy. Such curricula should take account of the changing educational levels of future generations of older people, while reflecting their different expectations of services for older people. Geriatric care is only one element and should not be overemphasized.

Opportunities for rehabilitation must be enhanced in many countries of the Region and made more easily affordable in some systems. Rehabilitation can be more cost-effective than keeping older people in hospitals. Homes offering care of the elderly should be based on the principles of maintaining their autonomy, self-esteem and civil status, and of gender sensitivity – women represent the majority of people living in such homes.

More appropriate health care and rehabilitation services could reduce the extensive drug use by older people. Where drugs are prescribed, the prescriber should consider the cost of the course of treatment, especially where elderly patients will have to pay for the drugs themselves. Containers should be labelled, and the size, shape, colour and appearance of tablets and capsules need to be appropriate for people who may have difficulties in taking medicaments.

> **HEALTHY AGING ON THE ISLAND OF SAMOS**
>
> A holistic support system for the elderly is being developed on the Aegean island of Samos which relies on community awareness among the islanders and cooperation between a number of different sectors. The aim is to ensure a better distribution of local resources and to provide a safe environment which promotes the emotional as well as the physical health of elderly people. The project will also benefit the tourist sector by promoting a healthy and safe environment to encourage elderly visitors to Samos, thereby generating income for the island which can later be ploughed back into improving services.
>
> A support centre for the elderly where medical records would be held is to be set up. Any request for care from an elderly person or his or her carer will be transmitted to the appropriate professional (for example, nurses, pharmacists, social workers, physiotherapists, etc.) together with the appropriate information from his or her records. Requests for care can be made manually or automatically anywhere on the island using telematics (e.g. via personal mobile telephones and automatic paging and locating devices).
>
> In Samos, carers are still generally people within the local community, family or neighbours. Initiatives such as "elderly-friendly" shops, hotels, and restaurants, etc. make life easier for older people, both locals and visitors, and their carers. Other changes on the island include improvement to paths and street surfacing, the provision of ramps and handrails to improve the mobility of the elderly, better facilities, and shaded rest areas.
>
> *Source*: Humphreys, P. *Healthy aging on the island of Samos. Networking for health.* Copenhagen, WHO Regional Office for Europe, 1996 (RHN Conferences Series, No. 4).

3.6 Dying in dignity

In many countries of the Region, dying is increasingly not a natural phase of life but a time people spend in social and emotional isolation in hospital. Although the major part of health budgets is spent on people in the last years of life, and specifically in the period immediately before death, a growing number of patients are now starting to seek low-technology treatment in order to be able to die in dignity. There is also a widening debate in many Member States about the influence people themselves have, or should have, over their own death, a question that raises a great many difficult ethical issues.

PROPOSED STRATEGIES

All people should have a right to a death that is as dignified as possible and one which respects their cultural values. This can be ensured if Member States endorse policies which enable people, whenever possible, to die in a place they themselves decide, surrounded by people of their own choosing, and as free from pain and distress as possible. The wishes of the individual should be at the centre of decisions about death.

Professional education needs to be strengthened in the area of palliative care. Professional carers should reflect intensively on the spiritual aspects of life and its terminal stages, so that they come to accept death more as a natural part of human existence. In addition, appropriate support should be offered to the family, friends and carers of dying people.

The work carried out in a growing number of hospices is noteworthy. In these institutions, the focus is on palliative care and pain management. Special attention is paid to a caring environment, giving priority to social interaction with the patients and to comforting them as much as possible.

Chapter 4

Preventing and controlling disease and injury

> Target 6 – Improving mental health
> Target 7 – Reducing communicable diseases
> Target 8 – Reducing noncommunicable diseases
> Target 9 – Reducing injury from violence and accidents

4.1 The overall burden of ill health

The Global Burden of Disease study, initiated by the World Bank in 1992 and conducted with WHO, attempted to quantify the burden of premature death and disability worldwide as expressed in disability-adjusted life years (DALYs), a composite measure of the burden of health problems in terms of premature mortality and years of life saved with treatment, adjusted for severity of disability. Data are available for the World Bank's standard regions of established market economies (EME) and the former socialist economies of Europe (FSE).[9]

The top ten causes of the burden of disease for EME and FSE, from the year 1990 and with projections to 2020, are shown in Table 1. It is significant that these are all noncommunicable diseases. The calculations do not take account of the burden on a nation's health resources of caring for people with these illnesses, nor of the burden on individuals themselves, their families and communities.

---

[9] The use of terms such as "established market economies" and "former socialist economies" is for the purpose of descriptive analysis only and involves no political implications of any kind.

Table 1. The top ten causes of the burden of disease for established market economies and former socialist economies

		% of total burden	
		1990	2020
1.	Ischaemic heart disease	9.9	11.2
2.	Unipolar major depression	6.1	6.1
3.	Cerebrovascular disease	5.9	6.2
4.	Road traffic accidents	4.4	4.3
5.	Alcohol use	4.0	3.8
6.	Osteoarthritis	2.9	3.5
7.	Tracheal, bronchial and lung cancer	2.9	4.5
8.	Dementia and other degenerative central nervous system disorders	2.4	3.4
9.	Self-inflicted injuries	2.3	2.4
10.	Congenital anomalies	2.2	1.0

Source: Murray, C.J.L. & Lopez, A.D. *The global burden of disease: a comprehensive assessment of mortality and disability from diseases, injuries and risk factors in 1990 and projected to 2020.* Boston, MA, Harvard University Press, 1996 (Global Burden of Disease and Injury Series, Vol. 1).

Data from Health in Europe, a report on the third evaluation of progress towards HFA in the European Region (1996–1997), paints the same picture, also emphasizing the predominant influence of noncommunicable diseases on premature death and disability. Nevertheless, communicable diseases in Europe still impose a considerable – and for some diseases and many countries an increasing – burden on people themselves and on the health system, although they are a smaller problem in terms of the absolute numbers of people seriously affected.

This chapter discusses four main categories of disease and injury, all of significant public health importance within the Region. These are mental health problems, communicable diseases, noncommunicable diseases, and violence and accidents. In each category, the health problems are analysed and public health strategies put forward for addressing them. In all cases, the striking feature is the commonality both of risk factors and of the approaches to tackling them and thus preventing so much illness and disability. This chapter should be read in conjunction with Chapters 5 and 6, as regards action by the health sector and other areas.

4.2 Mental health

It is difficult to be precise concerning the magnitude of the burden of mental health problems. One reason is that there are inherent culture-related problems with defining mental health, so comparing and interpreting trends in different countries is sometimes difficult. Data from the European Region as a whole indicate that the proportion of the population suffering from severe problems (as registered and reported by countries) varies from under 1% to 6%, with most countries in the range of 1–3%. According to World Bank and WHO calculations based on DALYs, three major psychiatric disorders – depression, bipolar disorder and schizophrenia – constituted 9.5% of the total burden of disease and disability in the EME and FSE in 1990.

Other problems with significant psychological manifestations include: Alzheimer's disease; other dementias and degenerative central nervous system disorders; alcohol and drug use and dependence; anxiety disorders; and sleep disorders.

At the other end of the spectrum of mental health problems, data on perceived health are difficult to generate and to interpret. Nevertheless, the differences in the proportion of people who assess their health as being good or very good tend to support an east-west gradient in health similar to that for other causes of mortality and morbidity.

Suicide is a common cause of death in adolescents and younger adults (responsible for as much as 15% of deaths in 15–24-year-olds), where it is often related to alcohol and drug use. It is increasing among the elderly, especially in the NIS and among men aged 85 and older. The average suicide rates in the NIS show a typical U-shaped trend from the 1980s to the mid-1990s, caused by the temporary improvement from the anti-alcohol campaign in 1985, the subsequent end of the campaign and the influence of the recent socioeconomic transition. Since the end of the 1980s, trends in the suicide rate have been declining in 26 countries (45.7% of the population), including 9 countries where increasing trends had been reversed since 1980: in 17 countries (44.8% of the population) suicide rates are increasing. No data are available for 8 countries.

Data show that suicide is strongly related to depression, and that the under-diagnosis and under-treatment of depression is an important background factor for high suicide rates. Suicidal and depressed patients are mainly in contact with general practitioners (GPs), but only in a minority of cases are they adequately recognized and treated.

Risk factors for mental health problems are increasing; these include unemployment and poverty; migration; political upheaval; growing tensions between ethnic and other groups (especially in major cities); increasing homelessness; rising substance abuse of various forms; loneliness and the breakdown of social networks; and socioeconomic upheaval and deprivation.

There appear to be marked differences in the prevailing doctrines of psychiatric care between countries in western and eastern Europe. Many countries in western Europe have attempted to reduce the number of inpatient beds and to adopt an approach based on the provision of care within local communities close to where patients live and (hopefully) work, although for various managerial and financial reasons this has been difficult to achieve fully. Ideally, such local care should offer mental health promotion and disease prevention services to local communities, as well as treatment near to the patient's own home in close cooperation with local primary care services. However, the Region still has over 100 very large psychiatric hospitals, or "asylums", almost all of them in the eastern part of the Region. Many of these are in poor condition and often provide inhumane and outmoded care.

TARGET 6 – IMPROVING MENTAL HEALTH

BY THE YEAR 2020, PEOPLE'S PSYCHOSOCIAL WELLBEING SHOULD BE IMPROVED AND BETTER COMPREHENSIVE SERVICES SHOULD BE AVAILABLE TO AND ACCESSIBLE BY PEOPLE WITH MENTAL HEALTH PROBLEMS.

In particular:

6.1 the prevalence and adverse health impact of mental health problems should be substantially reduced and people should have an increased ability to cope with stressful life events;

6.2 suicide rates should be reduced by at least one third, with the most significant reductions achieved in countries and population groups with currently high rates.

PROPOSED STRATEGIES

This target can be achieved through several broad and interrelated approaches. The stigma associated with mental health problems can be reduced by making them subjects of discussion rather than taboo. Individuals' and communities' ability to recognize problems, to cope with them and to prepare for and deal with other stressful life events can be developed through means such as advocacy, information and life skills training in school, work and other settings.

Health personnel and other care givers need to be better educated, trained and kept up to date in identifying and addressing risk factors, in using appropriate new tools to recognize mental health problems earlier and in treating them according to modern methods. A systematic training programme for family health physicians, to improve their skills in diagnosis and treatment of depression, can have a major impact on suicide (see box below). A new screening tool developed recently – "WHO wellbeing 5" – consisting of five simple questions, more than doubles the average success of GPs in identifying serious depression in a patient. This tool can also be easily used by family health nurses, for instance, to identify individuals who need referral to the family health physician.

Preventive, clinical and rehabilitative services need to be of good quality, with an appropriate blend of community- and hospital-based services addressing the problems of specific population groups, including minorities and disadvantaged people. Most of the large "asylums" that still exist in the eastern part of the Region need to be replaced by a well balanced combination of acute psychiatric hospital wards and community-based services; improving these two areas is a challenge for virtually every Member State in the Region.

Basic and applied research, including measures to investigate and act on the factors affecting people's understanding of mental health issues, should be enhanced in order to improve strategies for prevention and treatment.

Policy-makers in health and other sectors need to make decisions with particular regard to the root social causes and risks factors of so many of these problems, as well as to ensure a more appropriate resource allocation.

EDUCATION OF GENERAL PRACTITIONERS AND ITS IMPACT ON SUICIDE ("THE GOTLAND STUDY")

A project in the 1980s on the island of Gotland – a part of Sweden with a population of 60 000 and at that time in a state of societal transition with a high suicide rate – has given positive results. As a result of intensive education concerning depression and suicide directed at the island's GPs, referrals for depression, the number of patients in inpatient care, and the amount of sick leave due to depression all dropped by 50%. In the first three years after the education was implemented, suicides decreased by about two thirds (mainly in females with a history of depression and in contact with GPs); and prescriptions of antidepressants and lithium increased significantly, with an equivalent reduction in the prescription of non-specific sedatives. However, at the end of the three years, these effects faded and continuous education on the subject was therefore introduced during the 1990s, leading again to positive changes.

Today, there are few female suicides on the island. However, there are still a significant number of male suicides, most of them unknown to medical care. Attempts to improve the situation for male patients, too, are being made through the use of a locally developed symptom profile form, which helps identify the "atypical" masculine depressive syndrome. Continuous education will in future focus more on male suicides and the importance of engaging the mass media and other groups in society in the task of finding, supporting, protecting and treating depressive and suicidal men.

Sources: Rutz, W. et al. Prevention of male suicides: lessons from the Gotland study. *Lancet* **345**: 524 (1995); Rihmer, Z. Strategies of suicide prevention: focus on health care. *Journal of affective disorders*, **20**: 87–91 (1996); Rutz, W. et al. An update from the Gotland Study. *International journal of psychiatry in clinical practice*, **1**: 39–46 (1997).

4.3 Communicable diseases

Accompanying the political and socioeconomic transition of many central, eastern and newly independent states, the European Region is experiencing an alarming re-emergence of once-forgotten diseases like cholera, diphtheria, malaria, and syphilis. The incidence and mortality due to that old scourge, tuberculosis, is again increasing in many countries. HIV, a relative newcomer to eastern Europe, is now rapidly infecting its cities and regions (while the incidence of acquired immunodeficiency syndrome (AIDS) is falling in western Europe). The spread of all of these diseases is abetted by the economic crises and social upheaval afflicting these countries. The international migrations accompanying this period of economic and social strife have also contributed to the spread of diseases.

Efforts against communicable diseases can be directed towards eradication, elimination or control.[10] The shining example of success in disease eradication is smallpox, which was wiped off the face of the earth more than 20 years ago through a WHO-coordinated, worldwide initiative. Poliomyelitis is already similarly targeted by the World Health Assembly for global eradication by the year 2000.

The prerequisites for success in elimination and disease control include effective techniques; well defined strategies; good laboratory-based surveillance; planning; management; funding; and, in particular, the appropriate political will on the part of Member States. Strong technical support in selecting and implementing the required strategies can be given by WHO and the EU, UNICEF and other organizations and agencies; WHO can also contribute to ensuring the broad international teamwork that is essential in order to motivate all countries and coordinate their actions so as to obtain maximum benefit through a Region-wide, mutually supportive effort.

The coverage of communicable disease surveillance varies greatly in Member States, and only part of the estimated actual disease incidence is detected in the Region. Many laboratories now have only limited capacity and resources, and each Member State should analyse its need to make improvements in the standardization of definitions and laboratory methods, communication links, and training and supervision of public health personnel, in order to ameliorate its own and thus also regional communicable disease surveillance.

Poliomyelitis elimination in the Region is part of the global eradication initiative and entails strategies of high routine immunization coverage, supplementary mass immunization and enhanced surveillance. A coordinated campaign of supplementary mass immunization in pre-school children (Operation MECACAR, including Mediterranean and Caucasus countries and central Asian republics) has been conducted annually since 1995. This has been mounted in concert with bordering Member States in the Eastern Mediterranean Region, and in close cooperation with international organizations (e.g. UNICEF), NGOs (e.g. Rotary International), bilateral agencies (e.g. the United States Agency for International Development – USAID) and a number of other institutions and donor countries. Thanks to high routine immunization coverage and these special mass immunization efforts, endemic transmission has apparently been interrupted in nearly all Member States of the Region. The last confirmed cases of poliomyelitis in the Region occurred in January 1998 in Turkey.

Small numbers of cases of neonatal tetanus continue to be reported, but in only about four Member States each year. The bacterium infects the umbilical cord after birth, and the methodology to eliminate the disease consists of ensuring tetanus vaccination of women of childbearing age and the delivery of babies under hygienic conditions.

---

[10] See Glossary of terms (Annex 5) for definitions.

Measles immunization has had a positive impact on the incidence of measles infection and a dramatic impact on the number of deaths. In a few countries, very high coverage has been achieved and the incidence rate has fallen below 1 per 100 000 population. Despite these successes, many other countries are failing to meet the goal of elimination (by the year 2000) as specified in the regional HFA targets set in 1984. With few exceptions, failure to achieve this target in the Region is due not to a lack of resources but to a lack of commitment. Despite falls in the mortality and morbidity associated with measles infection, the disease still results in substantial health care costs, and measles elimination can therefore produce a clear net cost saving in developed countries.

Most countries of northern and western Europe have a very low prevalence of hepatitis B virus (HBV) infection, with less than 0.5% of the population being surface antigen carriers; incidence rates, too, are very low. However, the virus is highly endemic in some eastern European countries and NIS, especially the central Asian republics. Owing to under-reporting and the fact that at least 50% of HBV infections are asymptomatic, it is estimated that the number of people infected each year in the region may be close to one million. Of these, some 10% will become chronic HBV carriers and some 20 000 will die from liver disease.

All modes of hepatitis B transmission are found in the Region, including perinatal and child-to-child transmission, nosocomial infection of health care personnel and patients through unsafe injection and sterilization procedures, unsafe blood products, and traditional medical and cosmetic skin piercing procedures, as well as infection through percutaneous drug use and sexual transmission. Unsafe injections and medical procedures merit special attention because injecting drug use is increasing rapidly and hepatitis B, C and HIV infection are spreading widely among drug users and their contacts. At present, sexual transmission is one of the commonest routes for acquiring the virus.

Diphtheria was one of the diseases targeted for elimination by the year 2000. However, while the European Region experienced a substantial decline in reported cases in the 1980s (to a low of 855 cases in 1989), there was a major setback when a serious epidemic occurred in the NIS in the beginning of the 1990s. This was due to the collapse of previously effective immunization and surveillance programmes, a lack of effective booster immunization and other factors. A massive immunization effort to control the outbreak, involving all 15 NIS, was undertaken in 1994, 1995 and 1997, coordinated by WHO and implemented in close collaboration with the countries concerned and with assistance from UNICEF, International Federation of Red Cross and Red Crescent Societies (IFRC) and many other agencies and donor countries. The sharply rising epidemic curve was reversed, and the number of cases decreased to about 8000 in 1997. It is estimated that the immunization campaign may have averted more than 500 000 cases in total and more than 10 000 deaths from this disease.

During the 1970s and later, a few Member States had very low immunization coverage against pertussis in young children, while some others suspended use of the whole-cell vaccine until recently, resulting in increased incidence, complications and mortality. However, the disease has been progressively brought under control in many countries, and the availability of acellular vaccines may well provide a stimulus for even better control in those countries which are able to afford them. Elimination is difficult due to the variable efficacy of the vaccines and the role of older children, adolescents and adults in continuing transmission. There is clear evidence that pertussis remains a serious disease but is controllable by existing vaccines.

Surveillance of invasive *Haemophilus influenzae* type b (Hib) disease has been restricted to a few Member States. Meningitis, epiglottitis and pneumonia are the most serious manifestations. The cumulative incidence at the age of five years (before vaccine was available) has been estimated at around two per thousand children in the Region. With the implementation of routine immunization in early infancy and childhood, several Member States have dramatically reduced the occurrence of invasive disease. There is some evidence that high vaccination coverage decreases the circulation of the organism, as well as providing individual protection.

The reported incidence of congenital rubella syndrome has been steadily decreasing in recent years, although good surveillance has been limited to a few Member States only. The condition was previously targeted for elimination, but the lack of resources in countries in economic transition and the lack of political will in other Member States have led to failure to achieve that goal. The first imperative for elimination of congenital rubella syndrome is to protect women of childbearing age, and the second is to interrupt rubella transmission in young children.

Mumps is still a widespread disease in the Region, although it was previously targeted for elimination. In 1995, 33 countries reported some 340 000 cases; given the limited surveillance carried out, this represents a moderate decrease over the past ten years (more than one million cases were reported in the Region in 1985). Mumps is less infectious than measles, and transmission may be interrupted at relatively lower vaccination coverage levels. Nevertheless, the coverage targets for mumps match those for measles and rubella, as the MMR vaccine is used against all three. The cost–effectiveness of immunization against mumps justifies the inclusion of the disease in the targets.

Since the beginning of the 1980s, HIV infection and AIDS has been one of the greatest challenges for human health. Already in 1984 the Regional Office and the Member States started intensive health promotion campaigns to combat the new threat of HIV infection. The large-scale programmes quickly halted HIV transmission through blood transfusion and other medical interventions and subsequently led to reductions in transmission among men having sex with men, and later even in injecting drug users, in many countries. After 15 years of continued increase, AIDS incidence showed a declining trend in 1996 and 1997. Now, however, the Region is again facing a grave danger that HIV infection may spread quickly, this time in the NIS and some CCEE, as HIV infection is already spreading rapidly among injecting drug users in some cities of Belarus, the Russian Federation and Ukraine, thus introducing the infection on a wider scale in these countries.

Analysis of HIV incidence by age group and gender shows that in the younger age groups more women than men are affected. This calls for specific strategies to protect young women from infections, in particular through sex education and empowerment of girls and women. New therapies with a combination of drugs, including protease inhibitors, have become available, which drastically reduce the rate of progression of HIV infections; however, these drugs remain extremely expensive, and the final effectiveness of their therapy remains controversial.

In previous decades, the European Region experienced a steady decrease in the incidence of the main STDs such as syphilis and gonorrhoea, and until about 1993 they represented a fairly minor part of the Region's health problems. More recently, however, a very worrying new epidemic of syphilis has suddenly occurred, particularly in the NIS but also in some CCEE. Reported cases of syphilis are a more reliable indicator, but no doubt there have been similar increases in other STDs, too. There are many reasons for this development: lack of sexual health education in schools; limited acceptability and quality of STD clinics; unavailability or high cost of condoms; a sharp increase in travel; a change in cultural and social values – particularly among the young – and a marked increase in prostitution (as a result of the recent widespread poverty and rising criminality in the countries concerned).

The incidence of congenital syphilis decreased during the 1980s, so that by 1990 practically no cases were reported. In the past few years, however, with the exploding epidemics of syphilis and other STDs in adolescents and adults in some countries of eastern Europe, congenital syphilis has re-emerged and increased at an alarming rate. Incomplete surveillance hinders a good estimate of the current disease burden. The combined epidemics of STDs in the general population and of HIV infection among injecting drug users presents the potential for a rapid spread of HIV infection throughout many eastern European countries.

The resurgence of tuberculosis (TB) is a challenging problem in the European Region. Incidence and mortality rates are increasing in many eastern European countries, and the previous downward trend in western countries is now levelling off or being slightly reversed. The spread of *Mycobacterium tuberculosis* resistant to antimicrobial chemotherapy (often linked to inappropriate treatment) is worsening the situation. The resurgence is not so much linked to HIV infection, as due, in most cases, to the effects of poverty, including poor housing, malnutrition, and substance abuse. In addition, owing to the huge problems currently being faced by the health services in the eastern part of the Region, late diagnosis, insufficient diagnostic capabilities and lack of drugs often make treatment programmes ineffective for large numbers of people. A further complication is the fact that many countries are still not systematically following WHO's guidelines for the diagnosis and treatment of tuberculosis, particularly the directly observed treatment, short-course (DOTS) strategy. These guidelines provide for cheaper and more effective treatment, as well as reducing the risk of emergence of multiple drug-resistant TB strains.

Acute respiratory infections in children, mainly pneumonia, pose considerable problems in terms of illness and mortality, particularly in the more southern and eastern parts of the Region. Many such infections are due to *Haemophilus influenzae* type b (Hib) and *Streptococcus pneumoniae*. The future availability of conjugated vaccines could further aid the control of acute respiratory infections.

Diarrhoeal diseases, including sporadic cholera outbreaks following importation, are also a serious problem, particularly in the south-eastern countries in the Region. They exact a heavy toll in terms of illness and contribute substantially to infant mortality, causing much human suffering and entailing considerable costs for the health care system. Childhood mortality from diarrhoeal diseases in some NIS is up to 200 times higher than in western European countries. The disease agents are of different types and spread primarily through contaminated water or food, but also by person-to-person contact with other infected individuals.

Until the beginning of the 1990s, the majority of cases of malaria reported by countries in WHO's European Region were imported from other continents. The situation started to change dramatically at the beginning of the 1990s owing to political and economic instability, civil wars, massive population movements and large-scale development projects. *Plasmodium vivax* malaria epidemics are under way in Armenia, Azerbaijan, Tajikistan and Turkey. In addition, Tajikistan has experienced a *P. falciparum* epidemic. The epidemics have considerable impact on the malaria situation in neighbouring countries, and the number of cases imported into Kazakhstan, Kyrgyzstan, Turkmenistan and Uzbekistan has increased considerably in the past four years. As a result of malaria importation, sporadic indigenous cases have been reported from Kazakhstan, Kyrgyzstan and Uzbekistan. Constantly increasing international travel and population movements have also led to the importation of some thousands of malaria cases into other countries of the European Region. As a consequence of the high number of imported *P. falciparum* malaria recorded in western European countries, several deaths also occurred, and the malaria case fatality rate in countries providing reliable statistics ranges between 1.5% and 7%.

TARGET 7 – REDUCING COMMUNICABLE DISEASES

BY THE YEAR 2020, THE ADVERSE HEALTH EFFECTS OF COMMUNICABLE DISEASES SHOULD BE SUBSTANTIALLY DIMINISHED THROUGH SYSTEMATICALLY APPLIED PROGRAMMES TO ERADICATE, ELIMINATE OR CONTROL INFECTIOUS DISEASES OF PUBLIC HEALTH IMPORTANCE.

In particular:

Elimination of disease[11]

7.1   by 2000 or earlier, poliomyelitis transmission in the Region should stop, and by 2003 or earlier this should be certified in every country;

7.2   by 2005 or earlier, neonatal tetanus should be eliminated from the Region;

7.3   by 2007 or earlier, indigenous measles should be eliminated from the Region, and by 2010 the elimination should be certified in every country;

---

[11] For definitions of "eradication", "elimination" and "control", see Glossary of terms (Annex 5).

Control of disease

7.4 by 2010 or earlier, all countries should have:

- an incidence level for diphtheria of below 0.1 per 100 000 population;
- new hepatitis B virus carrier incidence reduced by at least 80% through integration of hepatitis B vaccine in the child immunization programme;
- an incidence level of below 1 per 100 000 population for mumps, pertussis and invasive disease caused by *Haemophilus influenzae* type b;
- an incidence level for congenital syphilis of below 0.01 per 1000 live births;
- an incidence level for congenital rubella of below 0.01 per 1000 live births;

7.5 by 2015 or earlier:

- malaria should in any country be reduced to an incidence level of below 5 per 100 000 population, and there should be no deaths from indigenously-acquired malaria in the Region;
- every country should show a sustained and continuing reduction in the incidence, mortality and adverse consequences of HIV infection and AIDS, other sexually transmitted diseases, tuberculosis, and acute respiratory and diarrhoeal diseases in children.

PROPOSED STRATEGIES

4.3.1 Diseases targeted for global eradication or elimination in the European Region

Poliomyelitis

Targeted supplementary immunization of high-risk populations, guided by surveillance findings, will be carried out in order to be certain that transmission has been interrupted in the Region – this will be done by implementing Operation MECACAR PLUS, which will continue at least through the year 2000. Current eradication efforts also include the establishment of a procedure to certify the elimination of indigenous poliovirus transmission from all individual Member States. The process of certifying poliomyelitis elimination has been initiated by establishing a regional certification commission and national certification committees in all Member States. The first group of countries will present the necessary documentation to the regional certification commission in 1998, followed by other groups of countries in 1999 and 2000. Surveillance must continue for many years past regional elimination, until global eradication is certified.

Neonatal tetanus

Elimination of the disease requires the organization of integrated immunization services for women of childbearing age and of hygienic obstetric practices in each high-risk area where the disease still exists.

Measles

The European Expert Advisory Group on Immunization has proposed a number of milestones for measles elimination (see box).

MILESTONES FOR MEASLES ELIMINATION

- by 1999, subregional workshops will have been held to assist countries in developing national plans for measles elimination; the WHO Regional Committee will have approved the operational plan for the Region;
- by 2000, each Member State should:
  - have achieved 95% coverage with the first dose of measles vaccine;
  - be implementing a high-quality surveillance programme to monitor disease incidence and the proportion of susceptible people;
  - have established a national measles reference laboratory;
  - developed a national plan for measles elimination;
- by 2003, all Member States should have implemented the necessary supplementary immunization strategies and appropriate surveillance activities;
- by 2007, measles elimination should be achieved in all Member States;
- by 2010, measles elimination should be certified in the Region.

The target age groups for campaigns and second doses will vary from country to country, because of differences in the epidemiological situation, programme implementation dates, coverage, and vaccination schedules. Member States and many international partners will need to make a strong commitment to progressing towards the target of measles elimination.

4.3.2 Control of communicable diseases through immunization

Hepatitis B

This disease causes more morbidity and mortality than any other vaccine-preventable disease in most of the Region, and incorporation of a vaccine against it should be among the highest priorities in national vaccination programmes. Universal immunization of infants is generally recognized as the basic strategy for long-term control of hepatitis B in areas with high and intermediate endemic levels. However, the routine immunization of adolescents would have a more rapid impact on the incidence of clinical hepatitis B than routine immunization of children. Further strategies include combined universal infant and adolescent vaccination, with particular emphasis on adolescent women, but this dual approach, while being highly cost-effective, needs the allocation of substantial resources.

Once a universal vaccination programme is in place, efforts to vaccinate people at high risk of HBV infection should not be abandoned. In addition to targeted immunization, transmission of the disease can be reduced among health care professionals by taking universal exposure precautions in hospitals and other health care settings, and among injecting drug users by avoiding the sharing of contaminated needles.

Diphtheria

The diphtheria toxoid component of currently available combination vaccines used for primary and booster immunizations is capable of controlling the disease and bringing it down to pre-epidemic levels, so that it would no longer be of public health importance.

Pertussis

All immunization schedules should include a three-dose primary course of pertussis-containing vaccine, preferably as diphtheria/tetanus/pertussis (DTP), administered before six months of age. The primary series should be reinforced by a fourth dose given before school entry. The need for additional booster doses should be assessed by individual national programmes. The few Member States with interrupted or incomplete pertussis immunization programmes have recently adopted the routine use of newly licensed acellular pertussis vaccines: this, along with improved coverage, should result in better overall control of the disease.

Haemophilus influenzae type b (Hib)

The proposed strategies are: (a) to extend laboratory-based surveillance to all Member States; and (b) to introduce Hib vaccination. The introduction of routine Hib vaccination will control invasive disease and could make it possible to envisage future elimination.

Congenital rubella

The congenital rubella syndrome could be eliminated from many countries in the Region and be better controlled in others through specific strategies. It is essential that high vaccination coverage be achieved in young children, as low coverage will result in an increased number of cases in older children and adults, possibly with more cases of congenital rubella syndrome. Countries introducing rubella immunization in young children should ensure that the vaccine is also used to protect non-pregnant females, including girls before puberty. In countries using routine MMR vaccine, the measles elimination strategy should be considered as the core of the programme.

Mumps

With expanded routine use of MMR vaccine, very low incidence levels will be reached.

4.3.3 Control of other communicable diseases

HIV/AIDS and other sexually transmitted diseases

A programme to respond to this situation must include the following components:

- providing frank information on how to prevent transmission of disease through safe sex practices and needle exchange programmes for injecting drug users, and building up people's ability to take vitally important decisions regarding their own behaviour;
- ensuring the wide availability of condoms;
- safeguarding blood safety through appropriate screening and testing of blood and blood products;
- ensuring effective treatment and case management of STDs;
- creating an environment conducive to safer sexual behaviour and drug use through legal, economic and other structural measures.

This will require emergency action to redesign all national programmes dealing with STDs in NIS and CCEE. WHO, the Joint United Nations Programme on AIDS (UNAIDS) and other organizations will have important roles to play in helping countries to implement innovative programmes and in ensuring that they have the necessary resources to carry them out. The health sector's task is to create a real understanding of the seriousness of the health and social impact of these diseases among political leaders in the affected countries.

With the introduction of enhanced control measures based on early case-finding and effective case management, and the development of primary prevention and appropriate surveillance systems, syphilis can be controlled. Targeted interventions, in the form of routine screening and treatment of pregnant women within antenatal services and active follow-up of women included in partner treatment, have proved to be effective and economical. Concerted efforts using modern STD control strategies would mean that adolescent and adult disease would be better controlled and congenital syphilis would no longer be of any public health importance, as it is now in some highly epidemic countries.

Tuberculosis

Measures against TB include:

- following a countrywide programme for TB control using WHO guidelines in every local community, based on the DOTS strategy – this requires a well organized primary health care service;
- case detection by sputum smear microscopy examination of TB suspects in general health services;

- standardized short-course chemotherapy for at least all smear-positive TB cases under proper case management conditions;
- regular uninterrupted supply of all essential anti-TB drugs;
- monitoring system for programme supervision and evaluation;
- special outreach services to migrants and displaced persons, the poor, people with HIV infection and other high-risk groups.

Acute respiratory infections

Current measures to reduce this problem include:

- nonspecific measures such as improving housing and nutrition, ensuring a smoke-free environment for infants and children at home and in institutions, and breastfeeding of infants to enhance immune and nutritional status;
- ensuring appropriate treatment following WHO guidelines by integrated management of childhood illness – this requires an effective PHC service;
- expanding the use of vaccination against Hib to more Member States (see above).

Diarrhoeal diseases

Actions to reduce the incidence of disease – and to alleviate the course of the disease once it has occurred – have been clearly established (see Chapter 5 for improvements in water supply and food safety):

- ensure safe drinking-water for every household in the Region;
- ensure the safety of all food products produced and sold in the Region – this includes safety throughout the food chain, from production to final preparation in the home;
- improve personal hygiene through services and education – this is still a considerable problem in large parts of the Region, where sanitation facilities are still quite primitive and personal hygiene not according to WHO guidelines;
- ensure the wide availability of oral rehydration salts (ORS) in all PHC services in the Region where diarrhoeal diseases in children are a serious problem: this includes proper training of PHC staff – and their training of families – and providing families with ORS packages to be kept in readiness in case of need (this requires a well organized family health service).

Malaria

To deal with the problem of malaria in Europe and curb the resurgence of malaria in central Asia and the Caucasus, a Region-wide strategy has been formulated, focusing on endemic countries and those most at risk and consisting of:

- establishment of a surveillance and early warning system for the timely detection of epidemics;

- strengthening of national capabilities for malaria case detection and treatment activities, through the training of general health personnel and the provision of limited stock of antimalarial drugs, and the reagents and supplies required for laboratory diagnosis;
- improvement of the technical capabilities of public health personnel at national, provincial and district levels to plan, supervise and evaluate malaria control activities, through refresher training and provision of up-to-date technical guidelines and scientific literature;
- reinforcement of public health services' capabilities to control malaria outbreaks and epidemics, through the provision of limited stocks of effective residual insecticides and spraying equipment;
- health education and information on malaria prevention, and promotion of community participation in malaria control activities;
- chemoprophylaxis of groups at risk, with particular emphasis on pregnant women (who are often already anaemic due to other factors).

The malaria control expertise that used to exist in different research institutes in the Region some 20–30 years ago is now reduced to only a few expert centres. An additional element of the regional malaria control strategy is therefore to ensure the continuation of a minimum number of WHO collaborating centres that can support control efforts in affected countries, and to prevent the introduction of the disease into further countries in the Region. In view of the financial difficulties faced by affected countries, considerable support will be needed from donor agencies to sustain such a Region-wide strategy.

4.4 Noncommunicable diseases

Noncommunicable diseases represent the greatest burden of mortality and morbidity within the Region as a whole and in every Member State. In the CCEE and NIS, in particular, noncommunicable disease rates are high and increasing.

The factors affecting an individual's susceptibility to developing noncommunicable diseases are genetic, biological, behavioural and environmental. Research now indicates that a person's genetic make-up is more important in determining the likelihood of developing certain diseases than previously acknowledged. None the less, the reduction and control of behavioural and environmental risk factors remains the cornerstone of action to reduce the incidence and alter the course of noncommunicable diseases. Risk factors such as smoking, alcohol, obesity, a fatty diet, lack of exercise, and exposure to stress can be linked epidemiologically to specific individual diseases. Collectively, they offer the opportunity for an integrated approach which can contribute to the reduction of several of the most important noncommunicable diseases (e.g. cardiovascular disease, certain cancers, chronic obstructive pulmonary diseases, mental disorders, and violence and injury).

The knowledge therefore exists to prevent many cases of noncommunicable diseases. In addition, screening and case-identification strategies allow for their detection and diagnosis across populations and within individuals. Treatment has also become increasingly effective for some conditions such as coronary artery disease. Lastly, rehabilitation remains an important component of disease management, for all conditions. Several noncommunicable diseases are considered in more detail below.

Cardiovascular diseases include both coronary artery and cerebrovascular diseases, and hypertension. As shown in Table 1 (see above), they are two of the top three main causes of the burden of disease, and are even more significant in the former socialist economies than in established market economies. They are the main cause of death at older ages. A significant number of sufferers are left with medium- or long-term problems such as reduced physical capacity, less favourable employment status, or psychological and emotional disturbances. Lifestyle-related factors such as smoking, poor nutrition, obesity and insufficient physical exercise play a key role in the development of cardiovascular diseases. Treatment for some conditions, particularly artery disease, is increasingly effective in reducing mortality and morbidity. New and less invasive procedures such as percutaneous transluminal angioplasty (PCTA) and stenting have made a significant contribution both to reducing the burden of disease and to assisting sufferers.

Cancer also demonstrates an east-west mortality gap among people under 65 years. Most CCEE had a continuous increase in cancer mortality among people aged 0–64 years until 1990, with some levelling-off since, attributable mainly to the stabilization or decline in lung cancer mortality. In western Europe, cancer mortality started to decline in the 1980s, to a level in 1997 about 9% lower than in 1980 (when standardized cancer mortality was around 92 per 100 000).

The single most important risk factor for cancer is smoking, which is responsible for about a third of all cancers in the European Region. Lung cancer mortality among women in the eastern part of the Region is lower than elsewhere, because of less exposure to tobacco smoking in the past. Diet, especially lack of fruit and vegetables and high saturated fat intake, is an important risk factor for certain types of cancer. Other risk factors include infectious agents (e.g. human papillomavirus for cervical cancer), hazardous industrial chemicals and occupational factors.

In women, breast cancer remains the most important cause of cancer mortality throughout the Region, and in western European countries up to one in twelve women will be affected, with incidence rates rising. There are limited opportunities for prevention; however, age-specific screening strategies using X-ray mammography have been successfully introduced in some countries, with a reduction in observed mortality. Such strategies have also been introduced to detect pre-invasive cervical cancer in many countries.

Overall cancer mortality has not fallen significantly, despite the considerable resources devoted to detection, diagnosis and treatment. Inadequate management of terminal cancer also remains a serious problem. For many people pain control remains poor, with unnecessary suffering reducing the quality and dignity of the final stages of life.

Diabetes is estimated to affect 25–40 million people in the Region. When not adequately treated, it may shorten the lifespan and have many serious adverse effects on health, such as blindness, kidney failure, amputations, acute blood sugar crises, etc.; it imposes a considerable burden on health services. Mortality from diabetes shows stable or decreasing trends in central and eastern Europe and in western Europe, but rising trends from an initially lower rate in the NIS, possibly due to the extremely high prevalence of obesity. Diabetes in pregnancy poses a major risk to the mother and child.

Since 1989, the WHO Regional Office and the European branch of the International Diabetes Federation have been jointly running a major effort – the St Vincent movement – that reaches out to virtually every Member State with an innovative approach to substantially reduce serious health problems for people with diabetes.

The prevalence of chronic obstructive pulmonary diseases in some countries is reported to be as high as 2–7%. These have a major impact on the quality of life, disability, health care costs and work absenteeism. Causative factors include smoking, air pollution and exposure to allergens in the home, work or natural environment.

Good oral health contributes not only to the quality of life but also to preventing several diseases and maintaining general good health. The priority given to prevention of dental caries, especially in children, in some countries means that oral health services now need fewer resources than previously for treating caries, thus releasing resources for oral health improvement of other target groups, e.g. the elderly.

THE VALUE OF PREVENTION IN ORAL HEALTH – THE EXAMPLE OF DENMARK

Some 20–25 years ago, Denmark had one of the highest rates in Europe of prevalence of dental caries in children. Since the implementation of systematic preventive oral care, oral health promotion, including effective use of fluorides, and a quality-oriented oral health information system, Denmark now has one of the lowest rates of caries in Europe as measured by the mean DMFT (decayed, missing or filled teeth), and the targets for oral health at ages 6 (50% of all children caries-free) and 12 (no more than 2 DMFT) were achieved as long ago as the mid-1980s. The achievements and the quality of oral health care in children have been documented by implementation of a case-based oral health information system. A comparable system for measuring oral health outcomes in adults has been recently designed for Denmark.

One of the most marked reductions in dental caries prevalence among children and adolescents may be ascribed to the implementation of population-based programmes and high-risk strategies. Consistent with primary health care principles, school-based oral hygiene instruction, fissure sealing and application of fluorides, health education, interdisciplinary health projects and activities involving the community have all been organized. Although this strategy was implemented within the frame of an established Danish municipal dental health service, the preventive principles are simple and can easily be adapted or transferred to countries whose dental health care systems are organized differently.

Sources: Petersen, P.E. Effectiveness of oral health care – some Danish experiences. *Proceedings of the Finnish Dental Society*, **88**: 13–23 (1992); Petersen, P.E. & Torres, A.M. Preventive oral health care and health promotion provided by the Municipal Dental Health Service in Denmark. *International journal of pediatric dentistry*, 1999 (in press).

Preventing and controlling disease and injury

Oral health status is age-related and varies tremendously among social groups in countries of the European Region. In a few of them, and especially in some regions within countries, there is a very low incidence of oral health problems, while in others, most notably in the more eastern part of the Region, dental caries and periodontal diseases are widespread. However, in no area of public health can such a major problem be so easily prevented through very simple methods.

TARGET 8 – REDUCING NONCOMMUNICABLE DISEASES

BY THE YEAR 2020, MORBIDITY, DISABILITY AND PREMATURE MORTALITY DUE TO MAJOR CHRONIC DISEASES SHOULD BE REDUCED TO THE LOWEST FEASIBLE LEVELS THROUGHOUT THE REGION.

In particular:

8.1 mortality due to cardiovascular diseases in people under 65 years should be reduced on average by at least 40%, particularly in countries with currently high mortality;

8.2 mortality due to cancers of all sites in people under 65 years should be reduced on average by at least 15%, with mortality due to lung cancer reduced by 25%;

8.3 the incidence of diabetes-related amputations, blindness, kidney failure, pregnancy complications and other serious health effects should be reduced by one third;

8.4 there should be a sustained and continuing reduction in morbidity, disability and mortality due to chronic respiratory diseases, musculoskeletal disorders and other prevalent chronic conditions;

8.5 at least 80% of children aged 6 years should be free of caries, and 12-year-old children should have on average no more than 1.5 decayed, missing or filled teeth.

PROPOSED STRATEGIES

The knowledge exists to prevent, diagnose and treat many noncommunicable diseases. The situation analysis indicates several cost-effective and high-quality strategies, both for public health and at the individual, clinical level.

(i) Broad public policy approaches should be adopted to deal with risk factors to health in an integrated way, tackling both behavioural and environmental exposure. This is a major challenge at national, regional and local community levels. Examples of such policies comprise incentives for prevention; educational programmes; transport policies; control of environmental pollutants, etc. (these sectoral areas are dealt with further in Chapter 5).

The health sector can also be specifically responsible for a broad intersectoral approach. The objective is to take a comprehensive approach to the most important behavioural and environmental risk factors, e.g. smoking, alcohol use, unhealthy nutrition, lack of physical activity. Such an approach offers the opportunity to combine intersectoral public policy initiatives with population-based and individual case-finding and management interventions to reduce the prevalence and impact of common risk factors (see below). WHO's countrywide integrated noncommunicable diseases intervention (CINDI) programme offers an important model for such a combined approach. The CINDI programme, established in 1982, aims to reduce the burden of these diseases on society by controlling their major risk factors; it is based on the implementation and evaluation of demonstration projects. Thanks to long-term collaboration between the now 24 member countries, a unique body of knowledge and experience has been built up of the prevention of noncommunicable diseases through integrated approaches at the community level. The most impressive results were achieved in Finland, with a 73% reduction in CHD mortality over a 25-year period (Fig. 4). One of the important factors contributing to this dramatic decrease is dietary change; the Finnish nutrition policy recommends increasing the intake of low saturated fat foods and vegetables (e.g. a free salad with meals contributes to doubling vegetable intake). Food and nutrition policies are needed in all Member States to help reduce high levels of premature mortality and morbidity due to noncommunicable diseases.

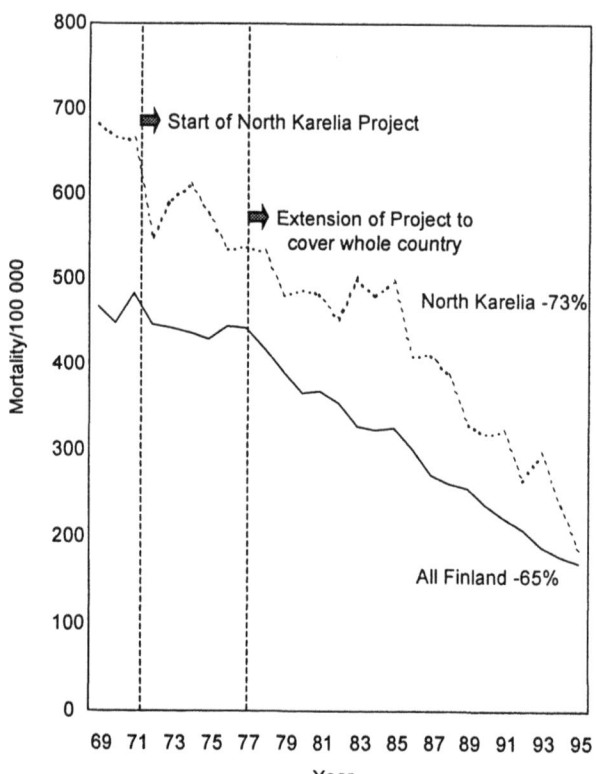

Fig. 4. Coronary heart disease mortality in all Finland and in the province of North Karelia 1969–1995 (Men aged 35–64)

> **THE HEALTH EFFECTS OF WALKING AND CYCLING**
>
> Regular walking is important in cardiovascular disease prevention and management. In a study of 9000 civil servants between the ages of 45 and 64, the 9% of men who graded their walking as "fast" experienced less than half the non-fatal and fatal coronary heart disease events of those who took no physical activity. Those assessing their walking to be fairly brisk had less than two thirds the rates of coronary attacks during the course of the nine year study. Similar findings on the value of walking and on the increased protection against disease as energy expenditure increases have been reported elsewhere. Research from Finland confirms such findings, suggesting that journeys to and from work by foot meet the intensity criterion of physiologically effective physical activity for fitness and health.
>
> A study among factory workers concluded that regular cyclists enjoy a level of fitness equivalent to that of individuals ten years younger. Another study found that those who cycled 60 miles a week from the age of 35 could add two years to their life expectancy. A Dutch study concluded that cycling as part of normal daily activities can yield much the same improvements in physical performance as a specific training programme.
>
> *Source: Road transport and health.* London, British Medical Association, 1997.

(ii) Preventive strategies should be population-based and, where appropriate, based on screening, e.g. for breast and cervical cancer. The objective of such strategies is to reach the entire population group at risk, with often initial contact through PHC-based population registers. Screening implies the use of a screening test; this is then followed, in those showing a positive screening result, by definitive examination, diagnosis and treatment.

(iii) Case-finding strategies, e.g. to identify hypertension should be based opportunistically on individual patient contact. These can be implemented by means of specific approaches to high-risk patients, again using PHC-based population registers. Such strategies may include the identification of risk factors; behavioural and lifestyle-based interventions; and management of conditions such as hypertension and diabetes.

(iv) For those with identified conditions, treatment services are essential and constitute an important dimension of the quality of their life. Diagnostic and treatment technologies have become increasingly effective, but strong interaction is needed between emergency, primary, secondary and tertiary care, with efficient processes for referral between the various levels.

These points are well illustrated by a number of diseases and conditions.

- *Cardiovascular disease.* As well as health promotion and disease prevention strategies to control and manage risk factors, strategies for treatment and rehabilitation are also required. These must start at population level, with emergency services providing rapid intervention for acute events, followed by rapid transfer to hospital and effective management (e.g. of coronary thrombolysis). Later treatment options include a range of medical and surgical interventions, with the latter increasingly being based on less invasive procedures (e.g. PCTA and stenting). Finally, well planned rehabilitation services are essential.

- *Cancer.* Diagnosis and treatment is also increasingly technologically based, with patients being offered more sophisticated combinations of surgery, radiotherapy, chemotherapy and, more in the future, immunotherapy. Palliative care and rehabilitation are essential elements of patient care services. New treatment modalities may also become available. Cancer management will increasingly be planned and delivered along integrated care pathways between primary, secondary and tertiary care, focused on centres of recognized clinical quality. Individual elements of patient care will be provided in accordance with evidence-based clinical guidelines. Services should be managed using agreed outcome-based quality indicators, supported by a comprehensive clinical information system.

- *Diabetes.* Comprehensive programmes for the detection and control of diabetes and its complications are required, with self-care and community support as major components. This means raising the awareness both of the general public and of health care professionals, with a strong component of training GPs and nurses in how to educate patients and their families to use essential techniques of self-care for diabetes management. Skilled and effective treatment at all levels of care must be clearly based on evidence and managed in terms of targeted outcomes at both population and individual levels. Such approaches have been shown to yield very significant improvements in clinical management and decreases in rates of complications. The key to success is the involvement of patients as well as their families in the planning and delivery of care, and in developing the competencies required for self-management. Ensuring that each Member State carries out a national programme as part of the St Vincent movement mentioned above will have a major impact on the health of people with diabetes in the European Region.

- *Oral health.* Individual oral health can be promoted by effective oral hygiene practices; improved dietary habits and the use of fluoridated toothpaste will almost completely prevent dental caries and periodontal diseases. Population-wide reduction of dental caries can also be achieved through appropriate fluoridation (of drinking-water, milk or salt) or through individual use of fluoridated toothpaste or mouth-rinsing with fluoride-containing liquid. Targeted, outcome-based monitoring and feedback are essential.

All disease control strategies require a sufficient evidence base, testifying to their effectiveness and efficiency, as well as to the accessibility and quality of the services provided. Such strategies should therefore be supported by a population-based health information system. This system should allow for:

- identification of the whole population and its epidemiology, i.e. mortality, morbidity, lifestyle and behavioural characteristics;
- planning and management of preventive and intervention strategies for noncommunicable diseases;
- management of individuals' involvement with such strategies, i.e. registering initial contact; recording the results of screening and case-finding interventions; monitoring follow-up; and recording outcomes;
- monitoring and evaluation of programmes in terms of their quality, focusing on the health outcomes achieved (see Chapter 6).

The sum total of interventions to deal with key individual health problems (e.g. cardiovascular disease, specific cancers) may best be thought of as health programmes, or specific areas for health improvement. An understanding of the basic health experience of the population, obtained from reporting and analysis of epidemiological and public health data, is a prerequisite for drawing up a programme. Consideration may then be given to the evidence supporting an appropriate balance of health promotion, disease prevention, therapy and rehabilitation (in both population-based public health policy and individual clinical management), and to appropriate care pathways and clinical guidelines. At the population level, this will emphasize the importance of multisectoral and interdisciplinary approaches; at the individual clinical level, it will allow for an evidence-based choice of interventions. Targeted, outcome-based monitoring and feedback, using agreed indicators will be essential at both levels.

4.5 Injury from violence and accidents

Intentional and unintentional violence has large human social and economic costs and is a major cause of death. In 1994 there were over 500 000 reported deaths due to accidents across Europe. Alcohol use is a major risk factor for all forms of violence and accidents. Other important factors are socioeconomic deprivation (e.g. poverty, poor housing, rundown urban areas), politically and socially unstable environments (e.g. war) and unemployment. Injuries and poisoning are the second most important contributor to the east-west mortality gap. Together with poisoning, accidents are the principal cause of death in young people.

Violence at home is in fact often a hidden problem, because it is seldom acknowledged by the victim or the perpetrators or included in accident statistics. Violence in the home is mainly, but not always, a gender-based problem; males are also victims. Twenty per cent of all women in Europe have been a victim of violence at least once in their lives, most often from someone they know, and – as mentioned in Chapter 3 – in industrialized countries domestic violence has been reported to cause more injury to women than rape, traffic accidents and muggings combined. Also important is the abuse of elderly people and people with mental health problems, particularly those in institutions. Socially motivated violence against refugees and ethnic groups is increasing. The extent of child abuse is also slowly being recognized (see Chapter 3): many countries in the European Region have in the past 20 years begun to document the incidence of sexual, physical and psychological abuse and its causes.

Accidents occur in a wide variety of settings (at work, home, school and leisure), with high associated costs. WHO has estimated that there are 80 million accidents requiring medical treatment in the Region each year.

The annual average incidence of reported road transport accidents involving injury is about 340 per 100 000 population in the EU countries. This is 2–3 times higher than the averages in the CCEE and NIS. The situation is reversed for mortality, with figures almost twice as high in the eastern part of the Region as in western Europe, indicating a much higher case fatality rate. Road accidents involving motor vehicles are the causes of injury and death that can be prevented most effectively. Measures include wearing good safety belts, improving the quality of roads and vehicles, enforcing adequate speed regulations, and reducing driving under the influence of alcohol.

THE COST OF TRAFFIC ACCIDENTS

In 1995, in the 15 member states of the European Union, there were around 45 000 reported deaths and 1.5 million casualties as a result of road traffic accidents. Taking into account levels of underreporting, it is estimated that the annual casualty total is near to 3.5 million. At current monetary valuations of the prevention of such deaths and injuries, these represent an annual loss of around 162 billion ECUs, which includes estimates for damage-only costs. This socioeconomic cost is around twice the entire budget of the European Union; accounts for 97% of the cost of all transport accidents; exceeds the cost of congestion or the environmental effects of road traffic; and causes greater lost productivity than even lung cancer. Efforts to reduce the number of deaths and injuries need to be all the greater because they have to outpace the likely increases in vehicular mobility resulting from economic recovery and growth in cross-border activity across the Single Market. Currently there is a sevenfold difference in risk between Member States where the risk is highest (Greece) and lowest (United Kingdom).

Source: A strategic road safety plan for the European Union. Brussels, European Traffic Safety Council, 1997.

Play areas for children represent an accident risk mostly because of the poor design of equipment and surfaces. Older children, however, often choose to play in more risky and unsupervised surroundings such as streets, wasteland, building sites, railway tracks, canals and rivers, and neglected safety measures in these areas can lead to serious injury and deaths.

Other relevant causes of injury from accidents are accidental poisoning, alcoholic poisoning, and sporting and leisure activities.

TARGET 9 – REDUCING INJURY FROM VIOLENCE AND ACCIDENTS

BY THE YEAR 2020, THERE SHOULD BE A SIGNIFICANT AND SUSTAINABLE DECREASE IN INJURIES, DISABILITY AND DEATH ARISING FROM ACCIDENTS AND VIOLENCE IN THE REGION.

In particular:

9.1   mortality and disability from road traffic accidents should be reduced by at least 30%;

9.2   mortality and disability from all work, domestic and leisure accidents should be reduced by at least 50%, with the largest reductions in countries with current high levels of mortality from accidents;

9.3   the incidence of and mortality from domestic, gender-related and organized violence and its health consequences should be reduced by at least 25%.

Preventing and controlling disease and injury

PROPOSED STRATEGIES

As for the other problems identified in this chapter, the strategies for addressing violence and injury are based on:

- knowledge about and surveillance of risk factors;
- public policies to address these risk factors, with particular attention to alcohol consumption and the reduction of social and economic inequity;
- no social and political tolerance for spousal, child and ethnically focused physical and sexual abuse, with appropriate legislative support;
- intersectoral action involving the political, legal, health and transport sectors;
- appropriate and integrated gender- and ethnic-sensitive prevention, care and rehabilitative strategies implemented primarily within primary health care;
- focused strategies where epidemiological information identifies major problem areas (for example, former army barracks, urban centres);
- research on the forms, determinants and impact of violence and injury, as part of the continued improvement of strategies for prevention, care and rehabilitation;
- advocacy and educational activities in places where young people gather (e.g. sports facilities, bars, school and work premises);
- public health advocacy and the provision of information concerning risks and preventive strategies;
- education and training of health personnel;
- monitoring and evaluation, including that of the impact of processes and strategies;
- establishing social networks;
- architectural design of neighbourhoods;
- in-depth treatment of the victims of family violence – who otherwise risk becoming the next generation of perpetrators.

4.6 Disasters

Emergency situations result from natural and man-made or technological disasters (e.g. earthquakes, nuclear accidents, chemical explosions and spillage); in addition, complex emergencies are the result of political, economic, social and institutional collapse, due to civil war, for example. All represent a significant challenge for public health.

Over the past ten years the European Region has experienced a significant increase in violent, complex emergencies, involving war or civil war. The disintegration of the former Yugoslavia provided the largest, tragic example, but in 1992, for instance, there were nine other conflicts within the European Region. Fortunately, the situation has significantly improved since then.

These emergencies have posed great demands for a rapid response in the form of resource mobilization and the provision of humanitarian aid. A large number of organizations – the Office of the United Nations High Commissioner for Refugees (UNHCR), UNICEF, WHO and other United Nations organizations, the EU, the Red Cross and many other NGOs – as well as many Member States have all been active in this work. While this has clearly revealed a need for better coordination and new methods of delivering emergency relief, much progress has been made on these issues through the large-scale operations carried out during the 1990s.

The WHO Regional Office also met this challenge and gained much operational, logistic and technical experience within the coordinated United Nations framework. More specifically, it has learned how to develop new technologies for future operations (emergency relief kits) and to design strategies for making a coordinated and efficient transition from emergency relief to recovery, rehabilitation and reconstruction.

PROPOSED STRATEGIES

Emergency preparedness

More efforts need to be made by countries to improve their emergency preparedness, establishing a supportive political, legal, managerial, financial and social environment for the coordinated and effective use of available resources. WHO can offer its accumulated technical expertise, guidance and training.

Humanitarian relief

When a major health emergency occurs, WHO's objective is to provide timely and appropriate humanitarian relief assistance, in collaboration with other agencies. Effective coordination of these activities within an overall United Nations response is effected by establishing close working relationships with other United Nations bodies, notably UNHCR, UNICEF and the World Food Programme (WFP). This assistance is based on a strategy of giving priority to assisting the government of the country concerned, by:

- becoming rapidly and credibly operational in the country
- assessing the public health situation
- providing technical assistance based on experience of tackling similar public health problems
- coordinating the health-related activities of the many NGOs present in emergency situations.

In addition, WHO has now gained experience of providing a range of individual public health programmes in areas such as water supply and sanitation, immunization (with UNICEF), and physical and mental health rehabilitation. Medical and surgical supplies and equipment are also provided, within the limits of the resources available, when there are clear indications that they are needed.

Rehabilitation and reconstruction

Later, when the emergency phase is over, WHO works with international development bodies such as the World Bank, the EU and the UNDP, to support, rehabilitate and reconstruct health services, emphasizing the PHC approach within the context of the HFA policy, as well as to provide special groups with essential health services. In addition, there is increasing awareness that health can be an effective vehicle for promoting dialogue and reconciliation and for building and promoting peace. Much recent experience has been gained in this area, for example in Bosnia and Herzegovina.

Although these activities are focused on assisting individual countries, some regional approaches are necessary in both emergency preparedness and response: these include coordinating with other international agencies (the International Atomic Energy Agency, in particular) concerning nuclear and chemical emergencies; providing a perspective for policy and implementation consistent with WHO's global policies and in consort with other international agencies; and coordinating with other United Nations humanitarian bodies on needs assessment and global resource mobilization.

Chapter 5

Multisectoral strategies for creating sustainable health

> Target 10 – A healthy and safe physical environment
> Target 11 – Healthier living
> Target 12 – Reducing harm from alcohol, drugs and tobacco
> Target 13 – Settings for health
> Target 14 – Multisectoral responsibility for health

Health results from the biological starting point of the individual and from activities involving most sectors of our society, as well as the population as a whole, through individual and collective decisions and actions. The choices people make are governed by external factors – which include their individual biological and genetic make-up, the physical environment, their socioeconomic circumstances and living conditions, as well as various political and cultural attributes – and the extent to which they have been empowered and given the capacity to make individual choices that will enhance health. Fig. 5 below provides a conceptual framework for analysing the various determinants and their interaction in creating health.

As introduced in Chapter 2, differentials in income and in access to education and employment are closely linked to differences in health and the quality of life between countries and between socioeconomic groups. Chapter 3 went further to demonstrate that socioeconomic circumstances alone do not determine health. Health results from the interplay of health determinants, life events and individual choices. Being poor means that people are at a disadvantage when it comes to making choices and coping with stressful life events. Chapter 4 focused on the prevention and control of diseases and their "immediate risk factors".

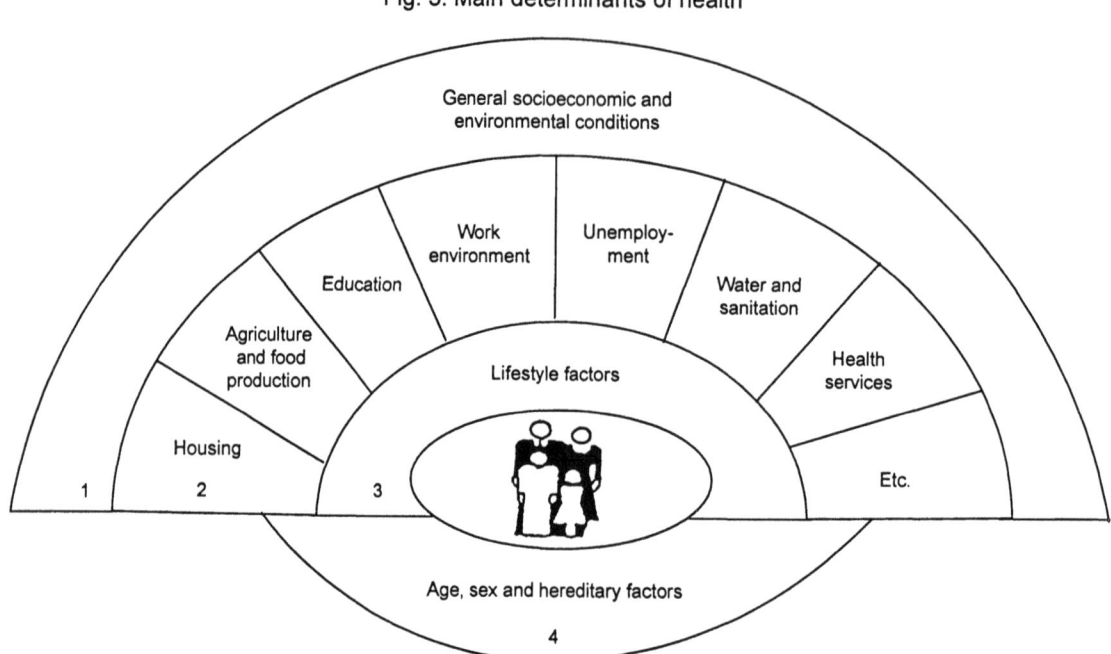

Fig. 5. Main determinants of health

Source: Dahlgren, G. & Whitehead, M. *Policies and strategies to promote social equity in health*. Stockholm, Institute for Future Studies, 1991.

This chapter provides the policy basis for dealing with the biological endowment for health and taking multisectoral action to create sustainable health and development by:

- tackling the physical and socioeconomic determinants of health;
- making it easier for people to make healthy choices;
- reaching out to empower individuals, local communities and private and voluntary organizations in different settings for health, e.g. homes, workplaces, schools and cities; and
- encouraging all sectors to identify and achieve mutual gains in terms of health and economic development.

5.1 The biological basis of health

The breathtaking and rapidly expanding technology of the "new genetics" has the potential to revolutionize the way we conceptualize the prevention and management of disease, but it also brings with it significant moral and ethical dilemmas. The human genome is a key contribution to health, alongside lifestyle, the environment and health care. The genetic determinants of health tend to have their most marked effects in early and middle life, with a major contribution to infant and childhood mortality, chronic morbidity, and premature onset of common disorders. The improved knowledge and identification of genetic factors responsible for morbidity and mortality throughout life emphasize the importance of profound and thorough discussion of the ethical questions attached to this issue. The conclusions from this ethical discussion should then form the basis for a European strategy.

Genetic factors contribute significantly to infant and childhood mortality. With an average birth prevalence of around 40 per 1000 live births, about half a million children with serious congenital or genetic disorders are born annually in Europe and, with a mortality rate of 2.5 per 1000 live births, at least 25% of infant mortality in western European countries is attributable to congenital or genetic disorders. Strategies using genetic approaches for management and prevention are required to further reduce these rates.

The "new genetics" combines advanced molecular biology with the knowledge of inheritance gained through genetics research. Locating a gene on a chromosome and identifying its DNA sequence are critical steps in developing diagnostic tests for those who may have a defective copy of that gene. The "new genetics" will take this further, by enhancing knowledge both about normal gene function and about the mechanisms, at molecular level, of diseases caused wholly or in part by defective genes.

Research so far has focused on simple inherited serious genetic disorders such as cystic fibrosis, sickle cell disease and Huntington's disease. The majority of the genes concerned have now been identified, and direct testing for the specific mutations involved in many of these single gene disorders is possible.

Attention is now being paid to specific genes involved in common diseases of later life. Here, patterns of inheritance are less clear cut, possibly involving several genes, and environmental factors may play a major role. Such diseases include diabetes, cardiovascular disease, cancers, schizophrenia and Alzheimer's disease.

At the moment in the European Region there is clear inequity in access to the two components of genetic services:

- a clinical genetics service offering diagnosis, counselling and locally based support for individuals and families. The clinical team will normally be led by a specialist, supported by genetics co-workers with responsibility for coordinating local service delivery; and
- laboratory services, including cytogenetics and molecular (DNA) analysis.

Research and development is providing opportunities for further clinical advances in three main areas:

- Screening and testing. Within the next 5–10 years, an increasing number of tests for single gene disorders and for genetic predisposition to common disease will be developed, and population screening programmes may also increase. Testing of asymptomatic individuals for predisposition to common disorders will provide opportunities for lifestyle adaptations to minimize risk. These tests may also include detection techniques to enable earlier interventions to be made, before symptoms appear.

- Symptomatic testing. Genetic tests will increasingly be used in symptomatic individuals to confirm diagnoses with great accuracy.
- Novel treatment regimes. These would involve two types of intervention:
  - as the molecular processes of disease are elucidated, the identification of specific targets will facilitate more effective treatments through rational drug design;
  - specific gene therapy is also theoretically possible, although significant advances may take some time.

Intervention measures have so far been based on prenatal diagnosis, thus entailing the difficulties associated with consequent termination of pregnancy. In future, the development of pre-pregnancy diagnosis is likely to make the genetic services more ethically acceptable, providing an option to control the outcome of pregnancy from the outset.

PROPOSED STRATEGIES

This "new genetics" offers the possibility that by the beginning of the twenty-first century many fields of medicine will be utilizing genetic advances in their practice, as well as in research. This will have significant consequences for the organization, staffing and delivery of health services, and a number of ethical dilemmas will need to be addressed.

A shared European strategy for the development of genetics services based on HFA principles would allow for a collaborative international approach and the sharing of expertise and experience. Each country should assess its need for genetics services and develop a national policy for their development, based on the principle of rationalization of services.

In the development of such a policy there appear to be five key issues:

- addressing the considerable ethical issues surrounding the development of several services;
- developing awareness of the needs of the population, including the needs of ethnic populations, engaging the public in planning appropriate services, and making services responsive to public preferences;
- providing sufficient education for health professionals;
- ensuring equity of access by the population to genetics services, including high-quality genetic testing services at primary care level, and the availability of advice and referral from the primary care level to specialized services;
- improving the quality of services.

Any programme development in genetics should focus on those priority areas which might have a major impact on health. These would include the most common congenital and genetic disorders in Europe, such as cystic fibrosis, haemoglobin disorders, severe congenital malformations and Down's syndrome. Most of the common single gene disorders should be considered as part of ongoing European programmes within maternal and child health and disease prevention and control.

In addition, because of the great relevance of cardiovascular diseases for health in the Region, and because of the emergence of new evidence about the role of genetic determinants in this group of disorders, cardiovascular diseases might be used as a target for exploring the possible impact of genetic approaches in health promotion activities.

Information will be a key factor; the "new genetics" may be considered as fitting well into the framework of "information age medicine", in which information technology empowers consumers to take greater control of their own health care, enabling health professionals to act more in a support capacity, with emphasis on health promotion rather than on managing disease.

Several ethical issues will need to be considered during this period of rapid development, and it will be important to monitor and assess the ethical, scientific and social implications of genetic engineering, including cloning technology. Genetic knowledge must be applied with due regard for the principles of medical ethics, such as respect for human dignity, autonomy and justice. The principles and content of the Council of Europe's Convention for the Protection of Human Rights and Dignity of the Human Being with regard to the Application of Biology and Medicine and its Additional Protocol on the Prohibition of Cloning Human Beings are of the greatest importance and should be universally followed.

Cell cloning or gene cloning can be of great clinical value in the diagnosis and treatment of diseases; it should not be confused with reproductive cloning. Somatic cell gene therapy for people with medical conditions is ethically comparable to any other therapy, and research in this promising area should be encouraged. However, germ cell gene therapy, where there is an intention or possibility of altering the genes passed on to the next generation, should not be permitted in the foreseeable future.

Genetic screening and testing can be an effective aid to public health planning in any country, but it should not be compulsory. Genetic counselling should be made available, within the context of local options and beliefs, and should be as non-directive as possible. Confidentiality and non-discriminatory use of genetic data should be protected, whenever necessary by legal means.

There is a need for a declaration or code of practice dealing with the new ethical issues arising from the medical and public health applications of genetics. As a starting point for such a declaration, a preliminary statement has been proposed by the WHO Expert Advisory Group on Medical Genetics (see World Health Assembly document A51/6 Add.1).

5.2 Physical and socioeconomic determinants of health

Good health and wellbeing require a clean and harmonious environment in which physical, physiological, social and aesthetic factors are all given their due importance. The physical environment should be regarded as a resource for improving living conditions and increasing wellbeing. Human health depends on the availability and quality of food, water, air and shelter. Although the impact of the physical environment on health has been known for some time, public awareness of environmental hazards has increased in recent years. This is the result partly of new scientific evidence demonstrating the link between the physical environment and health, and partly of the increase in new and potentially hazardous technologies. On a general scale, policy actions known to promote a healthier environment include moves to encourage the use of more resource-efficient technology; the introduction of environmental taxes; the mobilization of consumers through information and the media; and support to NGOs as the instruments of change.

There is still considerable uncertainty about the impact of human activity on the environment, and consequently on people's health, in the future. The global response holds that preventing the environmental damage which may result from climate change is far better than attempting to cure it, regardless of how fast and how soon it might be happening. The message from the United Nations Conference on Environment and Development held in Rio de Janeiro, Brazil, in 1992 was that a fundamental policy change is needed to protect the global environment and achieve sustainable development.

Scientific evidence has played an important role in heightening people's awareness of the impact of socioeconomic determinants on health, both directly and through their influence on health behaviours and neuro-endocrine pathways. There is now substantial evidence to show that poorer socioeconomic groups are more likely to be exposed to health risks and to adopt harmful behaviour patterns than richer socioeconomic groups. In practical terms, there is still a long way to go to create a socioeconomic environment that is conducive to health and wellbeing, and in particular to tackle the underlying socioeconomic causes of ill health (see target 2). This section sets out some of the challenges for health present in both the physical and socioeconomic environments and suggests ways in which they might be tackled.

5.2.1 Physical environment

In strategic planning and programme implementation, there is a need to ensure continuing cooperation between the health, environment and economic sectors in order to keep the health risks due to exposure to pollutants as low as possible. Air, water and soil need to be viewed as parts of a single whole environment, and the shift of risks from one part to another should be avoided. Policies that protect the environment require investment in all sectors, in order to provide the institutional structures, human resources and capacity-building facilities needed to tackle pollution of air, water, and soil and specific issues such as radiation.

Environmental health risk is not distributed equally, either geographically or throughout society. It is the poor who usually suffer most from the consequences of pollution. There are therefore strong links between goals for environmental improvement and for reduction in inequalities.

A Region-wide political commitment to action on the environment and health was achieved with the adoption of the European Charter on Environment and Health at Frankfurt in 1989 and of the 1994 Helsinki Declaration on Action for Environment and Health in Europe, as well as with the establishment of the EEHC.

Resulting from the 1994 Helsinki Declaration, the Environmental Health Action Plan for Europe and national and local action plans provide the Region and its Member States with a solid and comprehensive technical basis for action. National environment and health action plans (NEHAPs) collectively comprise a strategy to prevent and control environmental health hazards in Europe. As of June 1998, more than 90% of WHO's 51 European Member States are developing or have developed NEHAPs, each country writing its own plan with its own set of priority actions. WHO and its partners work with the countries to stimulate developments, advise on methodologies and support implementation of the national action plans. An important part of this cooperation is the sharing of countries' experiences.

Air

There is a close relationship between air pollution and the risks of damage to lung function, respiratory illness and death from respiratory diseases. Some 30–40% of people living in cities in the Region are exposed to average concentrations of air pollutants that are above WHO or EU guidelines. Widespread exposure to air pollution from sulfur dioxide, particulate matter, nitrogen oxides and volatile organic compounds continues in the Region, particularly in its eastern part. Nearly 90% of total sulfur emissions originate from fuel combustion, primarily in the energy sector. Road transport is the major source of emissions of nitrogen oxide and volatile organic compounds. Such emissions are likely to increase, especially in the eastern part of the Region.

Acid deposition, particularly of sulfur and nitrogen, causes widespread damage to natural resources of environmental and economic importance such as forests, soils and bodies of water. The major human health hazard comes from the movement of metals: cadmium and mercury from soils to the food chain, and lead and copper from community water supply systems to drinking-water. Health effects include damage to the nervous system from mercury and lead; kidney damage from cadmium; and liver damage from copper. Allergies relating to different air pollutants are also an important health problem.

Drinking-water and wastewater

Outbreaks of acute disease occur across the Region as a result of microbial contamination of drinking-water (a cause of gastrointestinal disease) or contamination with nitrates (a cause of methaemoglobinaemia in children), pesticides or other chemicals. Over 100 million people in the

Region lack safe piped water. Outbreaks of waterborne infection result from inadequate treatment of sewage, discharge of manure, breakdown in treatment operations or contamination during distribution. Harmful chemical contamination is largely a result of accidents or improper design of the distribution system.

In many places water is seriously contaminated by waste, including metals and sewage. In rural areas, widespread agricultural use of pesticides and nitrates over many years has contaminated groundwater and rivers and led to eutrophication. These problems remain greater in the eastern part of the Region. Contamination of ground- and surface water may affect health by lowering the quality of sources of water for drinking. In addition to drinking, water is also used for irrigation, fishing and recreation. It is imperative to protect the water cycle in its entirety. Water shortages are a major problem in some southern countries, mainly owing to poor management of available resources when the economy is expanding, exacerbated by irrigation, industrialization or growth in tourism. The costs resulting from poor management of the water supply and managerial inaction are very high. Some damage may be irreversible, as in some instances of pollution or over-abstraction of groundwater.

In general, a smaller proportion of the population enjoys adequate sewage collection and treatment facilities than has access to safe drinking-water. Under-investment in sewerage relative to water supply leads to harmful contamination of water resources and reduces the health benefits from investment in water projects. Leakage from drinking-water supply systems creates a need for greater quantities of water, puts a burden on treatment systems (thus leading to recontamination) and encourages the use of poorer-quality sources. Defects in badly maintained distribution systems, as well as interruptions in supply, can result in contamination of the network.

Solid waste

Hazards to health exist when absent or inadequate waste collection and disposal services lead to microbial and chemical contamination of air, water, food or soil. Uncontrolled hazardous waste, contaminated industrial areas, and leaching from landfill sites pose toxic risks and call for concerted action to prevent contamination of groundwater or food with chemicals from loaded soils.

Solid waste production is increasing at a rate that has outstripped existing capacity for treatment and disposal in a number of countries. Average production of waste is one kilogram per capita per day, a figure that needs to be drastically reduced if sustainable development is to be achieved.

Radiation

Natural background cosmic and terrestrial radiation is the largest component of average human radiation exposure. Concentrations of radon in buildings situated over radon-releasing rock have tended to increase when house ventilation has been reduced in order to conserve energy. Occupational exposure to radiation occurs in medical care and in the nuclear power and other industries. With the exception of some countries in the eastern part of the Region, average annual occupational exposure is decreasing to a level of the same order as the total natural radiation dose.

Nuclear power production in routine operation contributes radiation doses to the general population several orders of magnitude lower than total doses from natural sources. Actual or potential exposure problems are therefore primarily concerned with the safety of nuclear power facilities, the proliferation of nuclear material and the safe disposal or storage of nuclear waste. Due to increased awareness of risks and heightened public opinion and demand, the use of nuclear power is currently declining in a number of countries.

Radiation accidents fall into two categories: large-scale accidents releasing radioactive material over wide areas, and leakage from intact facilities. The largest accident that has so far occurred in the European Region was the 1986 accident at Chernobyl in Ukraine. The accident led to widespread distribution of radioactive material resulting in considerable contamination of the food supply; a sharp increase in thyroid cancers; persistent and profound negative psychosocial stress for a large number of people; and considerable costs in terms of containment and clean-up of the reactor site and the immediate environment, as well as from long-term non-use of polluted land.

There is considerable debate about the possible adverse health effects of exposure to non-ionizing radiation emitted by the electronic and telecommunication industries. Although such radiation has been reported to be associated with some increased risk to health, the validity of the findings, the level of risk and causal mechanisms still remain uncertain.

Exposure to ultraviolet radiation increases the risk of skin cancer. With increased travel and tourism, and reductions in the ozone layer, such cancers have become more frequent.

TARGET 10 – A HEALTHY AND SAFE PHYSICAL ENVIRONMENT

BY THE YEAR 2015, PEOPLE IN THE REGION SHOULD LIVE IN A SAFER PHYSICAL ENVIRONMENT, WITH EXPOSURE TO CONTAMINANTS HAZARDOUS TO HEALTH AT LEVELS NOT EXCEEDING INTERNATIONALLY AGREED STANDARDS.

In particular:

10.1 population exposure to physical, microbial and chemical contaminants in water, air, waste and soil that are hazardous to health should be substantially reduced, according to the timetable and reduction rates stated in national environment and health action plans;

10.2 people should have universal access to sufficient quantities of drinking-water of a satisfactory quality.

PROPOSED STRATEGIES

Air

Changes in individual and collective consumer behaviour as well as changes in production methods are essential to improve air quality. Each Member State must ensure that standards and guidelines are evidence-based. Air quality norms should be set and emission levels regulated to comply with

WHO and EU guidelines on air quality. Fiscal action can be taken, through the introduction of emission charges or taxes to reduce polluting emissions. The best available technology should be used, and new technology developed, to reduce polluting emissions. Strategies should cover the impact on air quality of road traffic, energy production, industry, agriculture and domestic sources. Particular attention should be paid to the transport sector.

Drinking-water and wastewater

Policy measures to protect surface water and water sources include the adoption of regulations (and, notably, the implementation of EU directives on nitrates); investment in infrastructure, particularly in sewage disposal and treatment plants; urban waste water treatment; action on agricultural, community and industrial waste to protect water sources; fiscal policy to control pollution through product charges or taxes on fertilizers and pesticides; and emission charges or taxes on waste.

The supply of adequate quantities of safe drinking-water can be achieved through adherence to standards based on WHO water quality guidelines, investment in delivery systems, and cost recovery. Water sector legislation requires an overall water law or equivalent enactment to ensure that the various aspects are comprehensively addressed. A water convention for the Region will be submitted for endorsement at the Third European Ministerial Conference on Environment and Health (London, 1999).

SAFE DRINKING-WATER THROUGH USING NATURE'S SERVICES

Until recently natural purification systems in the watershed, from where New York's water comes, were sufficient to cleanse the water to required standards. But sewage, fertilizer and pesticides in the soil reduced the efficacy of the process to the point where the water quality no longer met the required standards. The city was faced with the choice of restoring the integrity of the watershed at a cost of US $1–1.5 billion or building a new filtration plant at the cost of US $6–8 billion. It was clearly a cheaper investment to buy land in and around the watershed so that its use could be restricted and the construction of better sewage treatment plants subsidized, than building a new plant. Not only was health protected, but money was saved and an ecosystem preserved.

Source: Chichilnisky, G. & Heal, G. Economic returns from the biosphere. *Nature*, **391**: 629–630 (1998).

Water, sanitation and waste are public services that are essential for the health and wellbeing of individuals and communities. Under-investment in, and poor management of, these utilities leads not only to financial waste but also to health and environmental deficits. Considerable investment is required throughout the Region, but more particularly in its eastern part, to extend the coverage of safe drinking-water supplies and to build new sewage collection and treatment plants. Investment is required not only for the benefit of countries themselves, but also to protect international rivers and enclosed seas.

Infrastructure pricing strategies include connection, usage and peak capacity charges, to encourage efficient use and make provision for cost recovery.

Groundwater is of special importance because in its natural state it is usually of relatively good quality and because pollution and over-abstraction often have very long-term consequences. Treatment and reuse of wastewater is generally achieved most readily where industrial wastewaters are segregated from domestic sewage. Reuse of treated wastewater helps to reduce demand on primary water resources. In addition, local collaboration between sectors, including agriculture and land planning, is needed to ensure the safety of drinking-water sources.

Solid waste

The vast majority of waste is currently deposited in landfills. Technological improvements should reduce such disposal to a minimum, replacing it by combustion, composting or recycling, which have a negligible adverse environmental or health impact in urban and rural areas. Wide-ranging and radical change in individual and collective behaviour is needed to reduce waste and improve waste management.

National and local measures should include regulating the discharge of waste; using the best available technology to manage waste; and introducing stringent fiscal mechanisms, such as landfill taxes, to reduce waste production and encourage recycling and cost recovery. Improved management of industrial waste treatment and integrated management of municipal solid wastes should be encouraged, for example by making reuse and recycling financially attractive.

International action is required to prevent illegal or inappropriate trade in waste between countries.

CASES OF DISPUTED TRANSFRONTIER MOVEMENT OF HAZARDOUS WASTE

The international nongovernmental organization Greenpeace has been monitoring the transboundary movement of hazardous waste worldwide since 1986. Some of these shipments disregard national regulations and international conventions on the transboundary movement of hazardous waste. A large part of the shipments find their way through regulations by the promise of recycling, while what in fact happens is that waste moves from producing countries to those with fewer regulations and where disposal of such waste is cheaper. This is a situation that the Basle Convention (on the Control of Transboundary Movements of Hazardous Wastes and their Disposal) should prevent.

Source: Stannes, D. & Bourdeau, P. ed. *Europe's environment – the Dobříš assessment*. Copenhagen, European Environment Agency, 1995.

Radiation

Safety standards for nuclear power facilities are in place, but they need to be better implemented throughout the Region, using the best available technology and supported by European solidarity and strengthened information networks and capacity-building at the national and local levels. The medium-term use of nuclear power at the highest available level of safety, and with public support, should be assessed in the light of efforts to reduce air pollution from fossil fuels, pending the development of renewable sources of energy. Information on disaster plans and disaster preparedness should be widely communicated to the public.

To improve communication links among and within Member States and the relevant international bodies, such as International Atomic Energy Agency (IAEA) and WHO's global Radiation Emergency Medical Preparedness and Assistance (REMPAN) network, the Regional Office has established a project office associated with a national centre of excellence, in order to further enhance the capacity for preparedness and response in this field.

New research initiatives are necessary to evaluate recent studies concerning the health effects of non-ionizing radiation and to identify areas which require further investigation. The development of technologies which produce less emissions should be pursued and promoted.

In many countries, better construction codes and building guides need to be devised in order to achieve low radon concentrations in new buildings. Stricter implementation of safety standards and investment in safer new technology should reduce the occupational exposure of health care providers and their patients.

5.2.2 Social and economic determinants of health

Health is highly sensitive to socioeconomic circumstances, even in the most affluent societies, and therefore to socioeconomic policy and action. The main determining factors include income, education and employment. Some researchers attribute more than half of all illness to these underlying determinants. Even in low-income countries, health status can be improved if these factors are tackled. Changes over time in the health status of disadvantaged groups are a powerful indicator for assessing the success of socioeconomic policies.

> **IMPROVING HEALTH AT LOW COST: INVESTING IN SOCIAL DEVELOPMENT**
>
> Low income and fiscal constraint need not be barriers to improve the health status of the nation. The case of Sri Lanka, a poor country in the South East Asian Region, is instructive, also for European countries. Over decades, health has been improved at faster rates than in some richer neighbouring countries by implementing a development plan for all major sectors of the economy, reaching into every home: free education for both genders, subsidized housing, clean water supply and drainage systems, improved physical access to health care through subsidized public transport and an improved road network, and provision of a social security net for the poor through income transfers and food subsidies.
>
> *Source*: Kumaratunga, C. *Improving health at low cost: lessons and challenges from Sri Lanka*. (Address delivered at the Asian Development Bank seminar on "Health in Developing Asia: Seizing the Opportunities", Geneva, 28–30 April 1998).

Income distribution

Absolute income levels determine the poor health associated with poverty. Relative income differences, irrespective of social class, are related to the gradient in ill health and mortality that stretches across all levels of the social hierarchy. As income differentials widen, the risk of ill health widens. Social class differences in health are seen at all ages, with lower socioeconomic groups having greater incidence of premature and low birth weight babies, heart disease, stroke, and some cancers in adults. Risk factors, including lack of breastfeeding, smoking, physical inactivity, obesity, hypertension and poor diet, are clustered in the lower socioeconomic groups.

Income distribution is important not only for health but also for social cohesion. Societies in which there are high levels of income inequality also tend to have higher levels of violent crime. Deprivation leads to stress and economic hardship, reduces people's ability to fulfil roles, and contributes to psychological ill health. Income inequality must, however, also be looked at in the wider perspective of the extent to which social goods (e.g. free education) are available to lower income groups.

Socially cohesive societies are those with well functioning institutions and developed civic communities. With reduced income inequality, people can form and participate in social networks across society and through a variety of social organizations, purposes and activities. A sense of moral collectivity and social purpose remains important. When inequalities increase, social divisions become deeper.

Societies which pursue more egalitarian policies often have faster rates of economic growth and higher standards of health. The cost of inequality is a cost incurred for no economic benefit, but one that imposes a substantial economic burden and reduces the competitiveness of the whole society.

PROPOSED STRATEGIES

- Policies to ensure more equitable distribution of income and wealth, such as progressive tax systems, are an important element, as are social security benefits to specific age groups or low-income families. Giving more income to low-income people who are starting families has been demonstrated to result in higher birth weight babies.

BIRTH WEIGHT AND INCOME

Low birth weight is a marker for indices of deprivation and represents accumulated risk factors. Even when compared with others in the same social class, people with reduced birth weight have a raised risk of physical ill health, including death from coronary heart disease and mental ill health, in adult life. Birth weight is also related to subsequent social circumstances, including adult occupational social class, across the birth weight distribution from childhood to early adulthood. A randomized controlled trial in the United States showed that for pregnant women in low-income families, continuing in the ordinary welfare system or receiving an additional 50% income support, the women receiving income support had significantly fewer low weight babies than women in the control group.

Source: Kehrer, B. & Wolin, C.M. Impact of income maintenance on low birth weight: evidence from the Gary experiment. *Journal of human resources*, **14**(4): 434–462 (1979).

- Policies that address income distribution should be complemented by those that guarantee free health care and education, as well as subsidized housing. Employment and social services are also key contributors to improving health and reducing social exclusion.

- Measures to promote solidarity, civic participation and integrity, and pluralistic social and political networks can also contribute to better health through the development of healthy communities.

Employment

During the past ten years, unemployment has risen to new heights in Europe – about 12% in the EU, about the same in CCEE and about 6% in the NIS (from very low figures at the end of the communist era). Immediate forecasts are for little change in this situation.[12]

Both the quantity and quality of work have strong influences on many health-related factors, including income, social networks and self-esteem. Unemployment leads to psychological and physical ill health, as well as to labour market disadvantage. In a number of countries, the labour market has shifted away from secure unskilled or semi-skilled work, with on-the-job training, to work that requires a high level of pre-employment education and training, a development which has exacerbated youth unemployment, in particular.

Much has been made of the virtues for overall economic growth and development of a more flexible labour market, in which a high proportion of all jobs are temporary and a higher proportion of all workers are on short-term contracts or are formally self-employed freelance workers. Such job insecurity is associated with poorer health. Estimates of production costs, however, rarely take into account losses in health and the quality of life that are related to job insecurity.

Within employment, there is a clear association between grade of employment and mortality and morbidity, including sickness absence rates. The relationship is maintained even when allowance is made for other factors, such as level of education and housing tenure. The relationship seems to be explained by higher levels of work control, stimulation, and support in the higher grades. For example, a persistent mortality gradient has been found to parallel the job gradient inside the British civil service at Whitehall (see Fig. 6).

The health sector could begin by making itself a model work environment. Despite the fact that it employs a large section of the population, the health divide between different groups of health sector employees is rarely discussed but is very substantial, with low-paid personnel and assistant nurses, for instance, having several times higher risk of most diseases compared with doctors.

---

[12] *Economic survey of Europe 1998*. Geneva, United Nations Economic Commission for Europe, 1998.

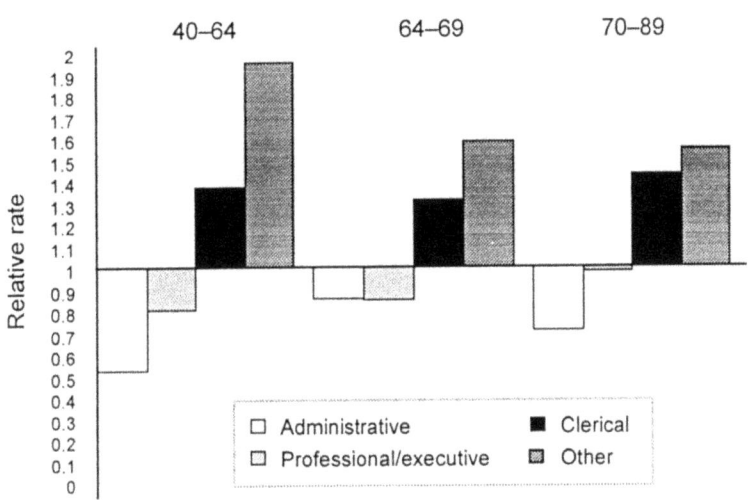

Fig. 6. All-cause mortality by grade, Whitehall men, 25-year follow-up

Source: Marmot, M.G. & Shiple, M. Do socioeconomic differences in mortality persist after retirement? 25-year follow-up of civil servants from the first Whitehall study. *British medical journal*, **313**: 1177–1180 (1996).

If, as is being predicted in some quarters, years of working life are to be compressed into a briefer period in future, new ways will have to be found whereby people can participate in society outside of work, and more people can share existing work.

PROPOSED STRATEGIES

- Securing adequate financial and social support systems for unemployed groups.
- Promotion of training and employment, especially of those who have experienced less favourable conditions in early life.
- Investment in secure employment to benefit health and long-term productivity.
- Inclusion in economic analysis of the stress of a high workload and job insecurity, in order to yield a better picture of the true outputs of economic activity.
- Flexible arrangements for sharing work.
- Alternative forms of social and community work, to avoid long-term structural unemployment.
- Adjustment of labour market policies to diminish the risk of discrimination on the basis of gender, age or ethnicity.

Education

Educational levels produce a gradient in mortality similar to that produced by social class. The material and cultural resources of the family have a major influence on a child's intellectual stimulation, encouragement and educational attainment. There is a strong social class gradient in educational qualifications. Children who have completed pre-university education or higher technical training or above have much better chances in health, as well as in occupation and income. Furthermore, education is a very strong predictor of making healthy choices. Higher and other forms of education foster innovation, which in turn sustains economic development.

PROPOSED STRATEGIES

- Nurturing of parental interest in and enthusiasm for education.
- Preschool education to help break the link with deprivation.
- Further improvement in the level of, and access to, education, more particularly of women but also of other disadvantaged groups.
- Allocation of economic resources to educational programmes according to clients' needs and the requirement of social equity.
- Setting higher educational standards and ensuring smaller class sizes.
- Training teachers and educating students in health issues.

EDUCATION – GIVING CHILDREN A HEAD START

In industrialized countries, the focus has changed over the years from raising overall literacy rates to tackling the educational disadvantages of growing up in poverty. The best known programme of this kind is *Head Start*, which began in 1965, targeting resources at half a million children in the poorest regions of the United States. Thirty years later, the programme is still running. A comprehensive package of services includes early education, immunizations, medical check-ups to detect hearing and vision defects, hot meals during the day, and social services and parental education/support for the families of the children.

Controlled studies have shown that the health of children participating in the scheme was better than those in control groups, as a result of better immunization, diet and dental health, increased access to services, and improved self-esteem and cognitive abilities. Longer-term results showed higher rates of entry into college and lower rates of arrest and teenage pregnancy among programme participants than in controls.

Source: Benzval, M. et al., ed. *Tackling inequalities in health – an agenda for action*. London, King's Fund, 1995.

5.3 Healthy lifestyles

It is sometimes wrongly assumed that just by providing people with information, they will automatically be able to make healthy choices. While more knowledge, information and health education is important, the evidence shows that decisions to adopt health-enhancing behaviour – for example, eating healthily, ensuring enough physical activity, and taking care of sexual health – are often constrained by the broader physical, social, economic and cultural environments which influence the choices that individuals, groups and local communities make. Furthermore, it is very often the poorest groups who adopt the most harmful health behaviour patterns, frequently with higher rates of smoking, alcohol consumption and drug use, since they suffer higher levels of stress in coping with inadequate income, poor education, and unemployment or job insecurity.

Therefore, one key focus for any programme must be to modify these environmental factors so that the healthy choices become the easy ones.

Since it is more often the better educated and advantaged groups that pick up health messages, this may further accentuate health differences and the social exclusion of vulnerable groups. Specially targeted health education and information programmes and competence-building for disadvantaged groups must therefore be a prerequisite for any successful initiative to promote healthy lifestyles.

Apart from enhancing individuals' competence in taking decisions about the type of lifestyle they adopt, the provision of information and education about health risks – such as eating unhealthily, smoking or drink-driving – leads, over time, to greater public support for policy measures to tackle tobacco and alcohol consumption and to promote healthy eating. Public awareness can be a powerful stimulus for change. Public demand for access to recreational activities, bicycle paths and better public transport has increased the possibilities of more active living. Public concern about the risks of environmental damage has led to greater demand for safe and environmentally friendly products. When this support is organized, as for example in consumer groups, people can be a powerful ally for health and a buffer against the forces that threaten it.

For the twenty-first century, Member States in WHO's European Region should build on the wide experience and substantial competence in dealing with lifestyles and health issues that has been gained in the past 15 years. The time has now come to build a broad alliance of Member States and organizations, in order to create the critical mass of forces that can bring about real change towards healthier lifestyles throughout the Region.

5.3.1 Healthy choices and behaviour

Healthy eating

Healthy eating concerns food and nutrition policies, food security, food safety, micronutrient deficiencies, and food and health choices. All WHO Member States endorsed the World Declaration and Plan of Action for Nutrition at the International Conference on Nutrition in 1992, and these provide a strategic framework for national food and nutrition policies.

Food security means that food is always available, accessible to all, nutritionally adequate in terms of quantity, quality and variety, and acceptable within a given culture. After the Second World War the main aim in Europe was to increase food security, especially animal products such as meat and milk. Some post-war policies were too successful, however, and in the 1980s the EU countries had massive surplus stocks of butter, meat and milk. These food policies have had a direct impact not only on health but also on the environment in Europe.

Epidemics due to newly identified pathogens have affected industrialized countries. In addition contamination, toxic materials, pesticides, animal drugs, agro-chemicals and the use of antimicrobials in animal feed all require constant surveillance. Global trade will make it more difficult to monitor these practices and related diseases, and it is therefore likely that more regulations will be required to protect food safety and health – but care will need to be taken not to make these regulations overly complex.

In the light of scientific findings on compounds, (antioxidants, flavonoids and phyto-oestrogens) which protect against the development of heart disease and cancer, for example, such diseases are sometimes called "diseases of vegetable and fruit deficiency". Deficiencies of other micronutrients also exist in certain European countries under certain circumstances: iodine deficiency diseases (IDDs), for instance, are endemic in Europe and afflict people in all but a handful of Member States. Iodine deficiency is the main cause of preventable intellectual impairment, in addition to goitre and cretinism. IDDs are targeted worldwide for elimination by the year 2000 (resolution WHA49.13). Increased consumption of folate is advocated in some countries to reduce the prevalence of babies born with neural-tube defects.

A diet characterized by a high proportion of high-fat dairy foods, fatty meats, salt and energy-dense foods containing sugars can pose an increased risk for noncommunicable diseases, such as cardiovascular diseases and cancer. This contrasts with the considerable intake of vegetables, fruits, bread, cereals and legumes recommended by WHO.

Excess body weight is an independent and increasingly important determinant of premature mortality. It can result from a high food energy intake induced by a high-fat, energy-dense diet and low physical activity, apart from genetic disposition. Excess body weight and obesity are widespread and increasing in most countries. Indeed, overweight and obesity are now so common that in many environments they are replacing more traditional public health concerns such as undernutrition and infectious diseases as among the most significant causes of ill health. The health consequences of obesity range from increased risk of premature death, particularly from cardiovascular diseases and some cancers, to several non-fatal but debilitating conditions that have a direct negative impact on the quality of life. In addition, obesity is also a major risk factor for chronic noncommunicable diseases (see Chapter 4) such as cardiovascular disease, hypertension and stroke, diabetes mellitus (type 2: non-insulin-dependent) and various forms of cancer. In many industrialized countries, obesity is also associated with various psychosocial consequences. A WHO consultation on obesity in 1997 made a series of recommendations for preventive measures.[13]

---

[13] *Obesity: preventing and managing the global epidemic. Report of a WHO consultation on obesity, 3–5 June, 1997.* Geneva, World Health Organization, 1998 (unpublished document WHO/NUT/NCD/98.1).

Physical activity

The health gains from moderate physical activity include enhanced mood and self-esteem, improved physical appearance and posture, and a substantial reduction in premature mortality, obesity, raised blood pressure, cardiovascular disease, non-insulin-dependent diabetes and osteoporosis. A 1990 national survey demonstrated that nearly one third of adults in England are living inactive lives, and that this proportion increases with age, a very worrisome fact which can make the elderly – women, not least – fall earlier below the minimum threshold of muscle strength needed for independent living. The Health Behaviour in School-Aged Children study, which covers 19 countries of the Region, found in 1993–1994 that between 60% and 90% of 11–15-year-old boys and between 40% and 80% of 11–15-year-old girls reported that they exercised vigorously two or more times per week.

The risk of physical inactivity is likely to increase with trends towards a more sedentary lifestyle. In some countries, levels of inactivity are so high that it is not possible to maintain a diet adequate in micronutrients without this leading to excess body weight.

Sexual health

Sexual relationships, which are an expression of communication, love and bonding, are an important aspect of adult life. While sexual health is conducive to human health and wellbeing, sexual activity can also be a risk to health. A considerable part of the total disease burden within the Region is estimated to result from unsafe sex; the current syphilis epidemic in NIS is one example, abortions due to unwanted pregnancies another. The rapid increase in HIV transmission related to drug use and the new STD epidemic in the eastern part of the Region also increase the danger of sexually transmitted HIV infection. Changes in sexual behaviour and attitudes and increased travel, poverty and unemployment and prostitution all contribute to the rapid increase in STDs.

TARGET 11 – HEALTHIER LIVING

BY THE YEAR 2015, PEOPLE ACROSS SOCIETY SHOULD HAVE ADOPTED HEALTHIER PATTERNS OF LIVING.

In particular:

11.1   healthier behaviour in such fields as nutrition, physical activity and sexuality should be substantially increased;

11.2   there should be a substantial increase in the availability, affordability and accessibility of safe and healthy food.

PROPOSED STRATEGIES

Healthy eating

A food and nutrition policy that guarantees food security in cereals, potatoes, vegetables and fruit is important for ensuring a healthy diet. The EU's reform of the common agriculture policy (CAP) should be influenced by health recommendations and dietary guidelines, since the new CAP will have a major impact on food consumption in the whole of Europe.

Public health specialists dealing with food safety and nutrition should strengthen their cooperation with those in other sectors (e.g. agriculture, the food industry, wholesalers, retailers and consumers) on developing food and nutrition policy. Moreover, food safety specialists and nutritionists should be encouraged to work more closely together on developing health targets as part of intersectoral food policies. This is increasingly important as the line between food safety and nutrition becomes more blurred because of the introduction of pre-cooked foods and functional, novel and special dietary foods, and the increasing use of food supplements.

Consumers have a vested interest in supporting the supply of safe, environmentally-friendly food of good quality which is nutritionally healthy. There is an opportunity to build stronger health alliances with the public interest groups working in the environmental and voluntary sectors. In an EU-wide survey carried out in 1996, consumer and environmental organizations were judged the most trustworthy sources of information by the public. There is a need to provide the public with more accurate and up-to-date information on food and nutrition.

HEARTBEAT WALES

This project was initiated in the early 1980s to help reduce the level of cardiovascular diseases in Wales. An innovation in its time and still a model of good practice among an extensive range of CHD risk reduction activities, this project *inter alia* included a broad range of actions to promote healthy eating. One example illustrates the approach – to reduce fat in meat, right through from the producer to the plate:

- farmers were encouraged to breed leaner animals
- slaughterhouses were encouraged to change their technology and leave more fat on the carcass
- butchers were encouraged to remove more fat and to promote the leaner cuts
- consumers were advised to buy leaner meat and to cook it in a healthier way.

These efforts were part of an integrated health promotion strategy which included, for example, policy development, community-based activities and advocacy work, embracing many hundred partners in private industry, NGOs and the public sector.

Source: Health Promotion Wales, Cardiff, 1998.

A healthy diet

There is scope for considerable health gain if people, especially those living in poverty, could have greater access to a diet rich in vegetables, fruit, unrefined cereal, fish and small quantities of good-quality vegetable oils, so that they consume a nutrient-rich diet lower in fat and energy density.

Consumers' food choices can be influenced in many ways. All links in the food chain can be used to produce food items that promote healthy eating and which are appealing, competitively priced and actively marketed. Pricing policies, too, can be used to promote a healthy diet. Educational programmes to convey the knowledge and skills required for growing, purchasing, preparing and eating a healthy diet should start in family and community settings and continue through pre-school, school and adult education. Professional education programmes can be provided for caterers, health care providers and others.

Remedying IDD is cheap, simple and always successful, provided it is done in a consistent and continuing fashion. Iodization of salt is the long-term solution, but initial measures such as supplementation of certain target groups may be necessary. A population well supplied with iodine is also better protected in the event of a nuclear accident releasing radioactive iodine.

PREVENTION OF IODINE DEFICIENCY

One of the ways currently recommended to prevent iodine deficiency is universal salt iodization. An upper limit of 6 g of salt per day is recommended by WHO. In some countries, such as the Nordic countries and the United Kingdom, the population get their iodine mostly from milk and milk products, since iodine is fed to cows. In the Netherlands, the salt in the bread made by the central bakeries is iodized, and in Iceland the population obtains its iodine mainly from fish.

Source: Department of Health. *Dietary reference values for food energy and nutrients for the United Kingdom.* London, H.M. Stationery Office, 1991 (Report on Health and Social Subjects No. 41); *Report on the addition of essential micronutrients to food.* The Hague, Netherlands Food and Nutrition Council, 1993.

SUSTAINABLE PRODUCTION FOR SUSTAINABLE CONSUMPTION – *FOOD FUTURE 21* IN SWEDEN

Growing and eating the right kind of food can reduce the risk of major diseases and simultaneously promote sustainable development and a healthy environment. For example, a futures study "Sweden in the year 2021" will, among other things, investigate the environmental impact of reduced intake of animal food. In this connection, a reference group has been set up with broad representation from different sectors, e.g. the food industry, retail outlets, transport organizations and consumers. As part of this study, the Swedish National Food Administration has worked out a diet with a reduced content of animal foods, compared with the current Swedish diet, in favour of increasing foods from plant origin. The diet consists of one third animal protein and two thirds vegetable protein and has a better balance of protein, fat and carbohydrates than the current Swedish diet. Meat and milk are partially replaced by more pulses, potatoes, bread, vegetables and fruit (at least one serving of pulses is needed per day to get enough protein). This new example from Sweden contains more vitamin C and fibre than the current diet but, although the content of zinc and iron is higher, there may be a slightly increased risk of deficiency, due to the fact that animal protein stimulates the uptake of iron; this could especially apply to women, children and the elderly. Nevertheless, this experimental diet will provide useful evidence on how the same recommendations for health and a sustainable environment are compatible and in unanimous agreement.

Food safety

In order to protect the consumer against unsafe foods, the emphasis in food laws has moved away from end-product testing and certification to risk assessment and food safety assurance programmes (e.g. using the Hazard Analysis and Critical Control Point (HACCP) system). The international approach to food legislation, in turn, is to move away from "vertical" standards that apply to specific foods towards "horizontal" rulings that apply to all foods. Labelling information should be comprehensive, correct and in the national language of the country where the product is sold.

Global trade makes it difficult to contain foodborne diseases, such as bovine spongiform encephalitis (BSE), within national borders. Most countries are therefore harmonizing their national legislation with international directives set by EU or the Codex Alimentarius, implemented by the World Trade Organization (WTO) to facilitate global trade. It is essential that public health professionals become more informed about international agreements on global food trade and take full part in the WTO Committee on Sanitary and Phytosanitary Measures. Only if public health specialists from the areas of both food safety and nutrition participate can they hope to influence future food policies.

Catering

The importance of providing and promoting healthy diets in all institutions, including those that are part of the health sector, is increasing. This is especially relevant where the number of meals supplied by public catering institutions (local authorities, civil service and school cafeterias, hospitals, meals-on-wheels, military establishments) is growing.

Retail outlets

Many services provided by retailers can greatly improve people's access to a healthy diet:

- large variety of fresh vegetables and fruits on sale;
- availability of small, reasonably priced food packs;
- unpackaged affordable vegetables and fruits sold singly for small households;
- free bus service to and from unserved areas, and wheelchairs and walking assistance for disabled people;
- loyalty cards or stamps that offer discounts on vegetables and fruits;
- home delivery service.

Physical activity

A substantial improvement in health is achieved by ensuring at least some 30 minutes of moderate-intensity physical activity, such as a sustained brisk walk, on at least five days of the week. The greatest gains are achieved among the sedentary who increase their walking. Strategies to increase activity should include transport, recreation and urban development policies. The aim should be to make use of a wide range of innovative approaches that together can succeed in inducing everyone to use their bodies more during the course of their daily activities. Also, good dietary patterns and physical exercise have a synergistic effect for good health.

Joint physical activity can strengthen family cohesion or other social networks and encourage respect for the environment. Housing and neighbourhood design can greatly promote walking as a natural, daily activity. Cars can be separated from bicyclists and pedestrians through adequate provision of cycle tracks and pedestrian sidewalks. Urban planning and settlement policies must ensure the preservation of open spaces that can be used for active recreation. NGOs, sports clubs, women's groups, scout movements, clubs for the elderly, etc., have important roles to play as part of a wide local community effort. Ensuring that areas where people walk, run or play are safe will require partnership with other sectors, such as those dealing with policing and law enforcement.

Sexual health

Sexual health policies and programmes must concern all segments of society, in particular adolescents and young people and susceptible groups such as sex workers and their clients, men who have sex with men, and injecting drug users. Information should be spread widely and communicated through education programmes carefully designed to develop respect for gender, to enhance life skills and communication skills, and to encourage the adoption of safer sex practices and acceptance of the family planning concept. Condom use needs to be actively promoted and marketed, in particular for young people, and condoms should be widely available, at prices everyone can afford – a particularly important concern in the more eastern part of the Region.

5.3.2 Reducing harm from alcohol, drugs, and tobacco

Tobacco

Tobacco use is the single most important risk factor for ill health within the Region. Fifty per cent of all people who smoke regularly will die from cigarettes, half in middle age (the most economically active period of life) and half in old age. Tobacco smoke increases the risk of many cancers, CHD, low birth weight, sudden infant death, allergies and a host of other health problems. In 1995, over 30% of adults within the Region were regular daily smokers. In the same year, cigarettes were responsible for 1.2 million deaths, with an average loss of 20 years of life expectancy. In the eastern part of the Region, 20% of all men aged 35 will die from a tobacco-related illness by the age of 69, twice as high a proportion as in the western part of the Region. By the year 2020, unless tougher measures are taken, cigarettes will be responsible for 20% of all deaths within the Region.

Tobacco products cost the world at least US $200 billion a year, cause untold suffering to individuals, families and friends; impose considerable costs on the economy; and are responsible for environmental degradation and fires. The significant economic losses are primarily due to premature cessation of productive life and the high costs of treating tobacco-related diseases. Failure to collect taxes on smuggled tobacco products (which are particularly prevalent in the eastern part of the Region, an area with scarce governmental resources) is also an important concern. One quarter of all cigarettes exported in the world are smuggled.

Alcohol

Alcohol products are responsible for some 9% of the total disease burden within the Region, increasing the risk of liver cirrhosis, certain cancers, raised blood pressure, stroke and congenital malformations. Although alcohol consumption reduces the risk of CHD, most of the reduction is achieved at levels of less than 10 g a day and is only relevant for people from their fifth decade of life onwards. At high levels of consumption, alcohol increases the risk of sudden coronary death. Furthermore, alcohol consumption increases the risk of family, work and social problems such as alcohol dependence, accidents (including fires), assaults, criminal behaviour, unintentional injury, violence, homicide and suicide, road traffic and shipping accidents, sometimes with extensive environmental damage. Between 40% and 60% of all deaths from intentional and unintentional injury is attributable to alcohol consumption. Alcohol-related harm is particularly high in the eastern part of the Region and responsible for a large proportion of the increase in cardiovascular deaths and reduced life expectancy.

Ninety per cent of the countries in the Region have an annual per capita consumption exceeding two litres of absolute alcohol (the level suggested by the evidence as the lowest population mortality risk). The cost of alcohol to society due to direct costs and lost productivity costs is estimated to be between 2% and 5% of GNP.

Illicit drugs

Illicit drugs include a wide range of substances which, because of their potential for harm, have been placed under the control of international conventions. Illicit drugs increase the risk of poisoning, dependence, psychosis, suicide, overall mortality and crime. The number of heavy drug users in the European Region is estimated to be between 1.5 and 2 million people. Drug use contributes to a further massive spread of HIV and hepatitis, especially in the eastern parts of the Region. Forty per cent of all AIDS cases in the European Region result from intravenous drug use. It is likely that a wider range of psychoactive drugs, some with potentially reduced risk of harm, will become available on the market, in addition to continued use of prescribed psychoactive medication.

In spite of substantial efforts to control drugs internationally and nationally, there are few signs of real improvement. Treatment and prevention approaches have become more sophisticated in recent years, with wider acceptance of substitution treatment for opiate-dependent persons. The evidence shows that societies which can afford an extensive network of services for drug users are successful in terms of reducing risky or straightforward health-damaging behaviour, as well as limiting antisocial and criminal activity among drug users.

> **TARGET 12 – REDUCING HARM FROM ALCOHOL, DRUGS AND TOBACCO**
>
> BY THE YEAR 2015, THE ADVERSE HEALTH EFFECTS FROM THE CONSUMPTION OF ADDICTIVE SUBSTANCES SUCH AS TOBACCO, ALCOHOL AND PSYCHOACTIVE DRUGS SHOULD HAVE BEEN SIGNIFICANTLY REDUCED IN ALL MEMBER STATES.
>
> In particular:
>
> 12.1 in all countries, the proportion of nonsmokers should be at least 80% in over 15-year-olds and close to 100% in under 15-year-olds;[14]
>
> 12.2 in all countries, per capita alcohol consumption should not increase or exceed 6 litres per annum, and should be close to zero in under 15-year-olds;
>
> 12.3 in all countries, the prevalence of illicit psychoactive drug use should be reduced by at least 25% and mortality by at least 50%.

PROPOSED STRATEGIES

Tobacco

Reducing tobacco consumption is one of the most important public health measures that can be taken to improve the health of the 870 million people in the Region. The 1988 Madrid Charter against Tobacco endorses the right of all citizens to a smoke-free and unpolluted environment. Strategies to achieve a tobacco-free Europe include establishing in law the right to smoke-free common environments, banning the advertising of tobacco products and identified brand-name sponsorships, and using revenue from taxes on tobacco to fund tobacco-control and health promotion activities. The Madrid Charter and the Action Plan for a Tobacco-free Europe provide the policy framework for action. Prevention strategies should seek to induce a fundamental change in society's standards, whereby nonsmoking becomes accepted behaviour. Gender-sensitive policies need to be implemented, since women are the target of the tobacco industries, particularly in eastern Europe.

As part of the development of a United Nations framework convention on tobacco products, the WTO should consider exempting tobacco products from free trade principles on the grounds of their serious consequences for health. Extending smoke-free environments at the workplace and in all places open to the public saves money and increase productivity. It sends an important cultural message that cutting tobacco consumption will enhance health and economic wellbeing.

---

[14] Or other age limits as appropriate to national legislation.

Increasing taxes on tobacco products raises government revenue and lowers tobacco consumption, particularly among young people. Tobacco taxes can be used to fund all tobacco control activities, including health education, research on tobacco control and support to health care. Using tobacco taxes is also an efficient way to fund sports and artistic events formerly sponsored by the tobacco industry. National and international public subsidies should not be used to promote the agricultural production of tobacco products.

If tobacco consumption and particularly that of children and young people is to be reduced, there will need to be a total ban on both advertising of tobacco products and identified brand-name sponsorship. Advertising through international media, including the Internet, should be regulated accordingly. Restricting the access of people under 18 years of age to tobacco products has been found to be effective in reducing illegal sales and in decreasing tobacco consumption.

1988 MADRID CHARTER AND TEN STRATEGIES FOR A SMOKE-FREE EUROPE

1. Recognize and maintain people's right to smoke-free common environments
2. Establish in law the right to smoke-free common environments
3. Outlaw the advertising and promotion of tobacco products and sponsorship by the tobacco industry
4. Inform every member of the community of the danger of tobacco use and the magnitude of the pandemic
5. Assure the wide availability of help for tobacco users who want to stop
6. Impose a levy of at least one per cent of tobacco tax revenue to fund specific tobacco control and health promotion activities
7. Institute progressive financial disincentives
8. Prohibit new methods of nicotine delivery and block future tobacco industry marketing strategies
9. Monitor the effects of the pandemic and assess the effectiveness of counter-measures
10. Build alliances between all sections of the community that want to promote good health

Source: It can be done, A smoke-free Europe. Copenhagen, WHO Regional Office for Europe, 1990 (WHO Regional Publications, European Series, No. 30).

Although the best available technology can be used to develop tobacco products with reduced tar and nicotine content, lower-yield cigarettes are not lower-risk cigarettes. More intensive smoking patterns from lower-yield cigarettes deliver high tar and nicotine levels and do not result in significant overall reductions in lung cancer rates.

> **THE CIGARETTE PAPERS**
>
> As a result of litigation in the United States the tobacco industry is increasingly being exposed to public scrutiny and made to pay for the damage caused. Tobacco industry documents, collected in a publication entitled *The cigarette papers*, make interesting reading. In the 1960s the tobacco industry wrote, "We are in the business of selling nicotine, an addictive drug". In the 1970s, the industry knew that "in most cases, the smoker of a filter cigarette gets as much or more nicotine and tar as from a regular cigarette". Partly as a result of these documents, the United States Food and Drug Administration acquired jurisdiction over cigarettes. Similar moves could be undertaken in Europe.
>
> *Source*: Glantz, S.A. et al. *The cigarette papers*. London, University of California Press, 1996.

A number of surveys show that some two thirds of current smokers report that they would like to stop smoking. Although it has benefits at any age, cessation before middle age reduces almost all excess risks. The use of treatment products for tobacco dependence, including nicotine replacement products, doubles the success rate of smoking cessation interventions. Unselective brief interventions by PHC providers are effective in supporting smoking cessation. They are one of the most cost-effective of all health care interventions, being 40 times as cheap as the median cost of 300 standard medical interventions. Training programmes need to be widely implemented for PHC providers, including nurses, physicians, pharmacists and dentists, and incentives offered for giving brief interventions in PHC settings.

The health professions in Europe have an important role to play in advocating for action against tobacco, supporting the reductions of smoking among their members and providing cessation services to current smokers who wish to quit. In this context, a very important element is the active support of this policy from all the national medical associations in Europe, acting through the European Forum of Medical Associations and WHO. Physicians, nurses and pharmacists are key players in providing advice and services to help people stop smoking, and the EuroPharm Forum (European Forum of National Associations of Pharmacy Owners/Pharmacy Associations and WHO) plays a key role in promoting this movement in the European Region.

Alcohol

There is substantial evidence from countries in WHO's European Region to demonstrate that significant health and economic benefits may be achieved by taking action on alcohol. The European Charter on Alcohol (Paris, 1995) outlines the main health promotion strategies, which include establishing and enforcing effective laws, taxing alcoholic beverages, and controlling direct and indirect advertising of alcoholic beverages. Health impact assessment of the industry is an important complementary strategy.

> **EUROPEAN CHARTER ON ALCOHOL – ten strategies for alcohol action**
>
> 1. Inform people of the consequences of alcohol consumption on health, family and society and of the effective measures that can be taken to prevent or minimize harm, building broad educational programmes beginning in early childhood.
> 2. Promote public, private and working environments protected from accidents and violence and other negative consequences of alcohol consumption.
> 3. Establish and enforce laws that effectively discourage drink-driving.
> 4. Promote health by controlling the availability, for example for young people, and influencing the price of alcoholic beverages, for instance by taxation.
> 5. Implement strict controls, recognizing existing limitations or bans in some countries, on direct and indirect advertising of alcoholic beverages and ensure that no form of advertising is specifically addressed to young people, for instance through the linking of alcohol to sports.
> 6. Ensure the accessibility of effective treatment and rehabilitation services, with trained personnel, for people with hazardous or harmful alcohol consumption and members of their families.
> 7. Foster awareness of ethical and legal responsibility among those involved in the marketing or serving of alcoholic beverages, ensure strict control of product safety and implement appropriate measures against illicit production and sale.
> 8. Enhance the capacity of society to deal with alcohol through the training of professionals in different sectors, such as health, social welfare, education and the judiciary, along with the strengthening of community development and leadership.
> 9. Support nongovernmental organizations and self-help movements that promote healthy lifestyles, specifically those aiming to prevent or reduce alcohol-related harm.
> 10. Formulate broad-based programmes in Member States, taking account of the present European Charter on Alcohol; specify clear targets for and indicators of outcome; monitor progress; and ensure periodic updating of programmes based on evaluation.
>
> Source: Alcohol – less is better. Copenhagen, WHO Regional Office for Europe, 1996 (WHO Regional Publications, European Series, No. 70).

The 1995 Charter on Alcohol and the European Alcohol Action Plan thus provide the policy framework to reduce the harm done by alcohol use. Increasing taxes on alcohol products reduces alcohol-related harm, particularly among younger people and heavier drinkers. A 10% decrease in per capita consumption will be matched by an approximately 20% decrease in male alcohol-related mortality and a 5% decrease in fatal accidents, suicides and homicides in the whole population.

Regulations are needed to control the alcohol content of beverages, to exclude claims making unwarranted connections between products and health, to control the packaging in which alcohol products are sold and to ensure that such packaging carries the necessary information (such as the ethanol content of the alcoholic beverage concerned). Alcoholic drinks masquerading as soft drinks that are designed and marketed to appeal to adolescents increase the risk of addiction and intoxication and should be banned. Advertising has a considerable impact on the use of alcohol products; restrictions lead to reduced alcohol consumption and less alcohol-related harm. If alcohol advertising is permitted, it should be restricted to print media and limited to product information.

Restrictions on hours or days of sale, and regulation of the number, type or location of sales outlets all decrease consumption. Raising the minimum legal drinking age can reduce alcohol-related road traffic accidents, as well as alcohol consumption and alcohol-related deaths. Responsible beverage service and beverage server training programmes, and greater legal liability for servers of alcohol, all help to reduce the number of accidents where alcohol is involved. The best available technology can be used to develop competitively priced high-quality alcoholic beverages with a low alcohol content.

Deaths from intentional and unintentional injuries, sudden coronary death and many social consequences of alcohol use are all results of acute alcohol intoxication. Targeted strategies to reduce the harm done by alcohol use should focus on reducing episodes of intoxication and separating drinking from the type of behaviour causing harm. Programmes to prevent alcohol consumption at the workplace are particularly important, as are actions and heavy sanctions aimed at preventing drinking and driving.

Brief interventions in PHC settings are effective in reducing alcohol consumption by over 25% in people with hazardous or harmful alcohol consumption. They are cost-effective, reduce health care costs and lead to improved health. Community intervention programmes can be effective in reducing traffic accidents involving alcohol, restricting under-age sales, promoting responsible beverage service and facilitating the adoption of local laws.

Illicit drugs

Intersectoral cooperation is needed at all levels between the health, social, education, law enforcement and justice sectors in order to come to grips with the health problems related to the use of illicit drugs. An integrated approach must be taken, reducing both supply and demand. Interventions on the supply side can restrict the availability of drugs. Increased emphasis should be placed on reducing the demand for drugs through educational programmes in community and school settings. Demand reduction programmes should be based on a comprehensive approach to all harmful psychoactive drugs.

Appropriate treatment and care services, matched to individual need, should be provided at community level to both drug users and their families. The aim of treatment is to enable a drug user to achieve a healthy and drug-free lifestyle over the long term. Specific harms associated with the use of illicit drugs, such as blood-borne infections, health problems, poverty, crime, violence and reduced productivity, can be lessened through risk containment strategies. The spread of HIV infection can be contained by targeting injecting drug users, organizing needle and syringe distribution and exchange, making condoms easily available, offering prescribed maintenance therapy, and expanding outreach services to less accessible populations. Such programmes call for some aspects of illicit drug management to be shifted from the criminal justice to the health care sector.

> **SWISS DRUG POLICY**
>
> In 1991, Switzerland introduced a drug policy comprising four strategic elements: (i) Law enforcement: Strict regulation or prohibition of certain addiction-causing substances and products. New legal instruments against money laundering and organized crime. (ii) Prevention: Convincing young people not to use drugs and offering programmes for groups at high risk of developing serious problems. (iii) Harm reduction: Protecting the health of addicts as much as possible during the addiction period, through appropriate measures such as needle exchange programmes, housing and employment programmes, etc. (iv) Therapy: A network of drug counselling centres and approximately 100 inpatient institutions (specifically designed to provide drug therapy with the declared goal of abstinence and social reintegration). About 14 000 drug users are following a methadone maintenance programme.
>
> Since 1994, the Federal Government has been supporting scientific studies of medically prescribed narcotics for severely addicted individuals. The main objectives are: to reach heroin-dependent people unable to profit from other forms of treatments; to improve the health and social status of participants; to reduce participants' risk-taking behaviour (including the risk of HIV infection); to compare results with those of other treatment approaches. Eight hundred patients (average age 30.8 years, average duration of heroin dependence 10.5 years, failure in other treatment approaches, with obvious social and health problems) are receiving heroin on prescription. The therapeutic programme includes on-site controlled injections (no take-home of injectables), comprehensive medical, psychiatric and social assessment, and a comprehensive care programme. Participation is voluntary. Some of the main results from the study (1995–1996) are:
>
> - somatic and psychological health significantly improved
> - illegal and "semi-legal" activities reduced (from 69% to 10%)
> - housing situation improved (homelessness from 12% to 1%, unstable situation from 49% to 21%)
> - employment rate in regular jobs improved (from 16% to 32%).
>
> With its fourfold approach, Switzerland has made remarkable progress in reducing the problems associated with drug consumption: there has been a noticeable reduction in AIDS and hepatitis infections, and in mortality from overdoses (drug-related deaths: 1992 = 419; 1997 = 241); open drug scenes have been eliminated; and the crime rate connected with obtaining drugs has been substantially reduced.
>
> Sources: *Swiss drug policy*. Berne, Swiss Federal Office of Public Health, 1998; *Evaluation of federal measures to reduce the problems related to drug use – Second synthesis report 1990–1996*. Lausanne, Institut universitaire de médecine sociale et préventive, 1997; *Programme for the medical prescription of narcotics – Summary of the synthesis report*. Zurich, Addiction Research Institute, and Berne, Swiss Federal Office of Public Health, 1997.

5.4 Settings to promote health

The previous section dealt with some of the issues related to individual choices and behaviour. This section recognizes that such choices are made in the everyday settings of daily life – the home, school, workplace and local community.

Taking a settings approach:

- focuses attention on where health is promoted and sustained (where people live, work, learn, play and receive health care);
- sets easily recognized boundaries of action;
- makes it easy to identify potential partners;
- provides the opportunity to observe and measure the impact of interventions for health gain;
- offers excellent potential both for pilot testing and as a "vehicle" for sustainable change in society.

Many different partners – engineers, architects, urban planners, retailers, people working in NGOs or the health sector, and many others – may influence the creation of a setting. Some constitute natural partnerships, others do not; but by learning to work together, the partners can make a major, innovative contribution to reaching the common goal of improving people's health. This section outlines some of the strategies for facilitating such joint decision-making and action in the settings of daily life.

Owing to pioneering developments in the European Region in the past ten years, the settings approach has acquired a new dimension as a strategy in its own right. Rather than just reaching out to the settings where people live, work and play, however, people must also be given a voice as individuals, groups and communities, to allow them more actively to influence the context in which they experience health. By taking control in the environment in which they live, people are also encouraged to take greater responsibility for their own health. However, to do so, they need efficient structures to manage.

Many different settings – not just those outlined below – are potential areas for action. It is important to tailor policies and programmes to reflect the interests of specific target group, and to consider the settings in which they may be reached. For example, using imaginative ways to provide information in settings such as video arcades, bars, clubs and prisons can be more effective in reaching a particular group (such as young men at risk) than working in more traditional settings.

Homes and neighbourhoods

The major health effects originating from poor housing are caused by lack of sanitation, damp, moulds, poor air quality, noise pollution, constructional deficiencies that predispose to accidents and damage during earthquakes, and unhealthy building materials including asbestos and lead-based paints. Lack of ventilation creates indoor air pollution, leading to respiratory allergies and illness. Individuals who live in households with smokers suffer particulate pollution two to three times higher than those who live in households with non-smokers. Total exposure to indoor air pollution will vary depending on the proportion of time spent outdoors, the ability of individual pollutants to enter the indoor environment, and the levels of pollutants generated indoors from cookers, paints, furnishings and building materials.

The housing stock in Europe varies considerably, from high-standard apartments and single-occupancy houses to low-standard multiple-occupancy blocks of flats where even basic sanitary facilities continue to be shared, when they are available. In general, the quality of housing is lower in the more eastern part of the Region. Homelessness is increasing throughout the Region, and all its health consequences, strongly related to poverty, remain an urgent problem.

Workplaces

Adults spend at least one third of their life at work, and the workplace has tremendous importance for their health.

It is estimated that 3–5% of GNP is lost because of the economic consequences of an unsafe and unhealthy working environment. Health problems at the workplace include accidents, exposure to noise and chemical hazards, ergonomic problems and stress. Moreover, the psychosocial work environment may be related to wider health problems outside the work sphere, such as heart disease and mental illness. Investment in better working conditions may lead to better health of employees and hence, to better productivity of firms.

Avoidance of work-related diseases and accidents is not the only major concern. Since the workplace is one of the few places where the adult population can be reached as individuals in a systematic manner, it is a major site for targeting adults with health promotion effectively, consistently and over time, and for building social networks.

Kindergartens and schools

There are great differences in educational programmes and institutions across the Region. In most countries, preschool establishments are not sufficiently viewed as educational institutions and therefore lack broad approaches to promoting health values, healthy behaviour and life skills. School health education programmes are often too traditional in their approach, giving students information on health issues but failing to use imaginative, interactive ways of providing education and training in mature decision-making, healthy behaviour, coping with stress, social relationships and other life skills.

Local communities and cities

Currently, some four fifths of the population in the western part of the Region and some two thirds of the population in the eastern part of the Region live in cities, which has direct implications for health. Cities require an extensive infrastructure for environmental health protection. Drinking-water supply, wastewater treatment and waste disposal technologies are all essential for healthy urban living. Urban shape, zoning strategies, noise levels and public amenities are important elements which can promote urban health and help to reduce stress, social dislocation and violence.

Within many urban environments, localized areas of deprivation exist, particularly in run-down city centres or chaotic peripheral zones, where environmental degradation and social exclusion go hand in hand. They are places of functional impoverishment with poor housing, insufficient equipment and inadequate social and recreational facilities.

A city's degree of social integration or social cohesion and its mortality patterns are closely interrelated. Interventions in high-risk groups have shown that the provision of social services and support improves the outcome in diseases such as myocardial infarction and the outcome of pregnancy in vulnerable groups and increases longevity in people with certain cancers. Socially underprivileged and disintegrated neighbourhoods contribute to people's sense of stress and frustration and inhibit the development of supportive networks.

Settings for people with disabilities

There will always be people who suffer impairment and disability, and demographic trends in the Region suggest that the number of such people will increase. The main causes of disability are locomotor disorders, sight and hearing problems, injuries and, increasingly, mental disorders, often associated with stigmatization and helplessness.

However, impairment and disability need not result in handicap. Too often, people with disabilities are made socially handicapped when they are denied the opportunities generally available to others. In many countries, the integration of people with disabilities is still far from satisfactory. Other countries show marked improvements in integrating disabled people.

Many children with disabilities continue to be inappropriately placed in institutions where they cannot fully explore their potential for development and independent living. Many adults with disabilities are often denied employment or given poorly paid jobs. Effective intervention is often weakened by a disproportionate allocation of available resources to highly specialized hospital technology. All too often, activities and services directed to people with disabilities receive only limited social and professional recognition.

> ### TARGET 13 – SETTINGS FOR HEALTH
>
> BY THE YEAR 2015, PEOPLE IN THE REGION SHOULD HAVE GREATER OPPORTUNITIES TO LIVE IN HEALTHY PHYSICAL AND SOCIAL ENVIRONMENTS AT HOME, AT SCHOOL, AT THE WORKPLACE AND IN THE LOCAL COMMUNITY.
>
> In particular:
>
> 13.1 the safety and quality of the home environment should be improved, through increased personal and family skills for health promotion and protection, and the health risks from the physical home environment should be reduced;
>
> 13.2 people with disabilities should have substantially improved opportunities for health and access to home, work, public and social life in accordance with the United Nations Standard Rules on the Equalization of Opportunities for Persons with Disabilities;[15]
>
> 13.3 home and work accidents should be reduced as specified in target 10;
>
> 13.4 at least 50% of children should have the opportunity of being educated in a health-promoting kindergarten, and 95% in a health-promoting school;[16]
>
> 13.5 at least 50% of cities, urban areas and communities should be active members of a healthy city or healthy community network;
>
> 13.6 at least 10% of medium- and large-sized companies should commit themselves to practising healthy company/enterprise principles.[17]

PROPOSED STRATEGIES

Homes and neighbourhoods

The home is the place where the core group of society, the family, should together discuss their health problems and agree on such things as a mutually supportive and healthy lifestyle. As mentioned in Chapter 3, a well trained, home-visiting family health nurse can be an invaluable support for the family in its health development efforts, as can a family health physician.

The home is also the physical environment in which people spend most of their time, and it should be conducive to health. Housing standards and building regulations should ensure the use of safe and suitable materials and proper building techniques; the availability of adequate lighting; a safe

---

[15] As contained in an annex to United Nations General Assembly resolution 48/96 of 20 December 1993.
[16] The health-promoting school includes education for health in the school curriculum and in the activities of school health services. A health-promoting schools network has been run jointly by WHO, the European Commission and the Council of Europe since 1992.
[17] Healthy company/enterprise principles include a safe working environment, healthy working practices, programmes to promote health and address psychosocial risk factors at the workplace, health impact assessment for marketed products, and contribution to health and social development in the community.

water supply; the provision of sanitation, heating and ventilation systems; resistance to damage from natural causes; proper insulation from outside noise; and a safe and continuous supply of energy for lighting, heating and cooking.

Housing policy must also be viewed in the broader context of urban and rural planning, covering such aspects as improvement of the housing stock, reversal of urban and rural decline, and shrinkage of areas of deprivation. Adequate health and welfare services, public transport, shopping and recreational facilities, and effective control of pollution and noise are essential for a healthy home environment. Policies should particularly aim to protect people who may be at risk of becoming homeless.

Those responsible for housing and neighbourhood design should look for solutions to counteract loneliness and strengthen social networks. Social networks and support improve health, increase social cohesion and make for safer communities. Housing and neighbourhood design should also pay particular attention to encouraging daily physical activity and make provision for groups with special needs, such as disabled and older people.

In many countries, the next two decades will entail rebuilding substantial parts of the housing stock – this offers the opportunity of introducing an HFA perspective into urban and regional development plans, thus laying a solid foundation for the future.

Workplaces

The aim should be not just to reduce exposure to risks, but also to increase employers' and employees' participation in promoting a safer and healthier working environment and reducing stress. One way forward would be for every workplace or enterprise to create a workplace-specific, HFA-oriented policy containing agreed targets and an action programme. This might be done by a health committee as a joint effort involving employers and employees, with support from the occupational health services. Programmes should address not only the prevention and treatment of accidents and disease but also broader issues of healthy lifestyles and environments. They will effectively promote a company culture that favours teamwork and open debate of problems, on the understanding that better HFA staff and better social relationships at work ultimately contribute to higher staff morale and productivity.

The principles of a "healthy company or enterprise" include:

- a safer working environment, including the prevention and control of physical hazards and screening for occupational risks and diseases;
- healthy working practices, such as a healthy eating policy in the canteen, and a nonsmoking policy;
- programmes to promote health at work and outside of work;

- initiatives to address psychosocial risk factors at the workplace, such as offering counselling; fostering supportive networks; induction and "mentoring" of new staff; supportive exit strategies; ongoing support at redundancy; and addressing major life events such as parenthood and bereavement;
- assessment of the health impact of the products marketed by the company; and
- contribution to health and social development in the local community, including outreach work with the community and building links with local unemployed people.

Kindergartens and schools

In addition to their role in imparting basic values, skills and knowledge, educational institutions should also serve to transmit and develop cultural identity and concepts of social responsibility, democracy, equity and empowerment. All children should have the right to be educated in a health-promoting kindergarten and school, as exemplified by the European Network of Health Promoting Schools.

In such institutions, education aims to provide the skills and action required for behavioural change, and not merely to transmit knowledge. Similar principles to those mentioned above for workplaces are also applied to institutions of learning. So in kindergartens and schools, teachers, parents and the children should be partners who together design, implement and evaluate programmes to enhance their basic health values, promote healthy lifestyles for themselves, prevent accidents and acquire basic life skills – all with technical support from the school health service.

Preschool facilities and the early classes of primary schools can promote health by laying down the ethical foundations and fundamental attitudes to support health, as well as by establishing healthy eating habits, personal hygiene practices, basic life skills, and social responsibility. Programmes for older children and adolescents can promote health through skills training and peer-led education on issues such as the use of alcohol, drugs and tobacco, sexual health, coping with stress, and social and parenting skills.

Lastly, involving schools in activities to promote health and support health care in the local community, for example by encouraging children to visit elderly people living alone or to act as advocates in nonsmoking campaigns, is an important way of generating greater understanding of the real problems people face.

Local communities and cities

Designing an HFA-oriented community health policy with health targets and an action programme, and monitoring and evaluating its implementation, is a vital component of work towards HFA, to be tackled on a properly planned basis by every local community, rural area and city in every Member State. The WHO Healthy Cities Network in the European Region (which has spearheaded a global initiative) now covers some 40 "WHO cities" and national networks in 25 Member States, involving a total of more than 1000 cities and towns in the Region which are committed to improving the health of their people.

The healthy city/healthy community concept involves the elected local council and representatives of major sectors such as health, education and social affairs, as well as the principal NGOs, the media and the local population. The local public health officer, and other public health professionals, have an important technical and leadership function in this work. For larger cities, one recommended approach is to break them into smaller sectors for planning and organization of PHC services, since that can ensure greater involvement of local groups and greater relevance of the action taken.

The urban infrastructure should allow a high-quality environment which will promote and protect the health of the inhabitants. So people and their living conditions should be the central consideration for town planning. Sustainable urban patterns can be achieved through balanced land use and the efficient use of space. The segregation of groups and individuals should be avoided as far as possible, and facilities and public spaces need to be accessible to all. Citizens can be encouraged to live peacefully together by promoting active interchange between generations and among ethnic, cultural and socioeconomic groups.

Promoting efficient transport management through urban road pricing, integrated public transportation, vehicle priority schemes, traffic calming, traffic bans in designated areas and parking controls can reduce air pollution, congestion, noise and accidents. Orienting urban renewal projects towards improving the quality of urban life, reducing the use of water, energy and materials and implementing programmes for separate waste collection, recovery and recycling can result in more sustainable cities.

Opportunities for people with disabilities

The health of people with disabilities can be improved if social and health policies create equal opportunities for people with disabilities, so that they can be fully integrated into the normal social and economic life of their community. People with disabilities must have every opportunity to enjoy family life, education, employment, housing, access to public facilities and freedom of movement. Action should be aimed at counteracting helplessness and stigmatization.

A public debate, based on information about the broad range of disabilities, is urgently needed in order to destigmatize impairment and disability and to raise awareness of the fact that, because anybody can be afflicted, disability is a matter of general societal importance. Policies need to include arrangements for monitoring the quality and appropriateness of health services for disabled people. Mass media campaigns, such as that on dyslexia in Sweden, show very promising results. Comprehensive, pluralistic approaches to the treatment of impairment or disability are more effective than single-track approaches.

Early intervention strategies should be applied, in order to secure compliance with specific support and treatment measures. Intersectoral coordination remains essential, in order to ensure training and placement, education, access to public transport and the creation of physical environments designed for use by all. Most important, disabled people themselves (and their organizations) must be guaranteed a major role in planning and making decisions about national and local community programmes to meet their special needs.

5.5 Multisectoral responsibility for health

As shown in previous chapters and in sections 5.1–5.4 above, healthy lifestyles can be promoted and healthy environments created only by mobilizing a large number of different sectors. An effective approach to health development therefore requires all sectors of society to be accountable for the health impact of their policies and programmes, and sectors other than health also to recognize the benefits of promoting and protecting health.

The health and wellbeing of a society is an expression of its socioeconomic and physical environments, of people's capacity to make healthy choices, and of the settings where they live. It is very clear that health does not arise from actions pursued solely by the health sector; rather, it is a manifestation of all public policies and how they individually, or in interaction with each other, promote or damage health. Until now, the business of promoting and protecting health has largely been recognized as the responsibility of those working in the health sector, across the entire continuum from prevention to care to rehabilitation. However, the fundamental message underpinning target 14 is the need now to generate more widespread action and accountability for health and awareness of mutual objectives in protecting health across all sectors.

There are two essential elements to achieving accountability for health; first, making a health impact assessment of any social and economic policy or programme likely to have an effect on health, and, second, enhancing public involvement. The importance of health impact assessment, beyond the environment sector, is still not generally recognized. On the contrary, most other sectors, apart from the social sector, do not perceive that they have a role in creating and damaging health.

TARGET 14 – MULTISECTORAL RESPONSIBILITY FOR HEALTH

BY THE YEAR 2020, ALL SECTORS SHOULD HAVE RECOGNIZED AND ACCEPTED THEIR RESPONSIBILITY FOR HEALTH.

In particular:

14.1 decision-makers in all sectors should take into consideration the benefits to be gained from investing for health in their particular sector and orient policies and actions accordingly;

14.2 Member States should have established mechanisms for health impact assessment and ensured that all sectors become accountable for the effects of their policies and actions on health.

Proposed Strategies

5.5.1 Achieving accountability

Effective mechanisms need to be established, including incentives and legislation as appropriate, to motivate all sectors for health-supportive action and make them accountable for the health effects of their policies and work. The health sector has the principal, but not sole, responsibility for "placing health higher on the political agenda", by providing the evidence base to raise health concerns and by making these known to government, all sectors, the public, political and business leaders. The health sector also should lead the way in formulating integrated policies for health and development, with clearly defined priorities, objectives and targets, reliable indicators to monitor progress, and transparent processes to search for common or converging objectives in other sectors (see Chapter 7).

If other sectors are to be motivated to act and be accountable for health, they should also provide the leadership whenever this is appropriate, and the health sector needs to recognize and support initiatives by other sectors which have a positive health impact. Such recognition can support the identification and creation of alliances for mutual gain. The health sector also needs to find ways of resolving potentially conflicting objectives between sectors while promoting and protecting the values of HFA, playing the role of advocate in highlighting the likely benefits of action for health by other sectors.

Accountability also rests on the leaders in government who create policy, allocate resources and initiate legislation – in the health sector, as in all sectors. Governments, national and regional parliaments and city councils should request health impact assessments of major legislation and policies. In all countries, measuring progress in socioeconomic development, in terms of recorded changes in the health status of the most vulnerable people is an essential element in achieving such accountability.

In much the same way as the Organisation for Economic Co-operation and Development (OECD) reviews economic and educational policies, WHO could act as an independent agent in reviewing or auditing, on request, national and regional policies. There are already examples of this, such as a review of the Finnish HFA policy and "health audits" in Hungary and Slovenia. As regards methodology, health impact assessments should be relatively simple and practical to implement, while sufficiently complex to recognize that health is influenced by socioeconomic determinants and policies in other sectors.

Measures to ensure that people are fully informed about health impact should be high on the political agenda in all countries of the Region. Public involvement can be enhanced through broad participation in health impact assessments, disseminating the results of assessments, and organizing public enquiries and hearings on the health impact of major projects.

National and regional parliaments and city and community councils can ensure that information is available and accessible by regularly reporting on equity in health status. Measures such as ensuring that all publicly listed companies report to their annual general meetings, and publish in their written annual report, statements about pollution or emissions during production, the health implications of the products, and health and safety in the workplace, can be an effective way of making the private sector accountable for its actions. The introduction of HFA values into professional guidelines for a wide variety of experts and managers throughout the economy could go far in encouraging accountability for equity and sustainability in health and development. Journalists, for example, have recently been developing ethical codes and professional guidelines on this basis.

NGOs at all levels are indispensable as agents of change, raising public awareness of health and environmental trends and their consequences and demonstrating alternative and sustainable economic and social systems.

5.5.2 Action for health by other sectors

This section is designed to open up a dialogue with other sectors on how they can promote health and how they stand to benefit from doing that. The various policy responses are intended as a first analysis, and the list is by no means exhaustive. Expanding the range of options (based on the mutual interests of health and other sectors) should be a major goal for the twenty-first century. The examples given build on the dual notion that the promotion and protection of public health should be essential criteria for the choice of policies and strategies in the economic and social sectors, and that other sectors often stand to further their own objectives by adopting these criteria.

Business and industry are becoming increasingly aware of the advantages of sound environmental and health practice. This has come about not just in response to the health sector but as a result of increased consumer demand for environmentally friendly and health-promoting production processes and products. Products are increasingly being priced according to their true cost, in other words including their cost to health and the environment. Consumers increasingly know what they are paying for, and are often willing to pay more for a product they know is safe and healthy and which has been produced safely.

THE VERONA INITIATIVE

In order to identify pragmatic ways to facilitate collaboration among the actors/partners decisive in the creation of health, the Verona Initiative was set up in 1998. The aim is to identify opportunities and threats to intersectoral collaboration and to create awareness of the possible impact of policy decisions on determinants of health. The "Verona Benchmarks" provide a framework for measuring countries', regions' and local communities' capacities to implement intersectoral collaboration in line with the HEALTH21 concept and principles. Three-year pilot projects are currently ongoing in Italy, United Kingdom and Austria. More countries, such as Finland, are likely to establish such demonstration projects.

Energy

The provision of sustainable energy is central to the activities of households and to economic production. The energy sector can invest in health and the environment by improving urban air quality and reducing emissions of greenhouse gases, acid deposition, and radiation and other accidents, and the sector can also invest in the health of its employees and of people in the immediate surrounding environment.

POLICY OPTIONS

- Incorporation of "external" environmental costs into energy prices to make them better reflect real market prices (especially in central and eastern Europe) and to help conserve energy. Use of economic instruments, such as pollution charges, taxes, and tradable permits.

- Open and honest discussion of risks and new strategies for energy production and use involving both technical experts and society at large.

- Energy policies favouring renewable sources of energy and setting limits on sulfur emissions from fuel combustion (switching to natural gas will produce less sulfur per unit of energy).

- Energy efficiency programmes, focusing on the operating efficiencies of power stations and energy distribution networks, and on energy savings in transport and household sectors.

- Action to reduce the environmental impact of the energy sector across borders, in line with the Convention on Long-Range Transboundary Air Pollution.

Transport

Efficient transport is required for movement and access of people and goods. The transport sector accounts for 7–8% of gross domestic product (GDP) in the EU. Road transport is one of the fastest growing markets for energy use in the European Region; in particular, the number of cars on the roads in the eastern part of the Region is expected to increase markedly in the future. A doubling of road transport for passengers and freight is likely between 1990 and 2010, unless special measures are taken soon. If current trends continue, carbon dioxide emissions from transport will increase by a further 25% between 1990 and 2000; relative increases will be even greater in central and eastern Europe. The road transport sector has a lead role to play in improving air quality, reducing noise and congestion (particularly in urban areas) and conserving energy. The social and environmental costs of transport have been put at near 5% in the area covered by OECD.

Road traffic accidents are a large and growing source of Europe's burden of injuries. Cars also increase people's risk of ill health in less direct ways: through increased physical inactivity; scattered communities where children cannot move independently; and infrastructure, such as roads, with a significant adverse impact on the quality of the environment.

> **INTERSECTORAL ACTION TO REDUCE TRAFFIC ACCIDENTS**
>
> In the early 1970s, Denmark had the highest rate of child mortality from traffic accidents in western Europe. A pilot project was therefore started in Odense, for a programme that now has an ongoing budget of approximately US $150 000 a year. Forty-five schools participated in an exercise carried out with accident specialists, planning officials, the police, hospitals and road authorities, to identify the specific road dangers that needed to be addressed. A network of traffic-free foot and cycle paths was created, and a parallel policy of traffic speed reduction, road narrowing and traffic islands was adopted. Following the success of the pilot study, the Danish Safe Routes to Schools programme has been implemented in 65 out of 185 proposed localities and the number of accidents has fallen by 85%.
>
> Source: *Walking and cycling in the city*. Copenhagen, WHO Regional Office for Europe, 1998 (Local authorities, health and environment series, No. 35).

POLICY OPTIONS

- A unified transport policy to manage private and public transport, favouring a reduction in petrol-driven road transport, limiting nitrogen oxide and carbon emissions from motor vehicles and imposing speed limits on roads.

- Fiscal policy, regulations, and research and development to reduce pollution and shift transport towards less polluting and more energy-efficient rail and water transport.

- Restructuring existing energy taxes on petrol and cars in line with their impact on pollution.

- Specific policies to protect consumers and prevent injuries, including cars and roads designed with safety in mind; alcohol policies to prevent drinking and driving; and programmes to ensure the health and skills of those working in the sector.

Industry

All countries need a viable industrial base – it is a prime source of goods, services, employment and wealth. Sustainable and profitable industrial activity is that which invests in health and in the environment and, through labour policy, in human development and wellbeing. Industrial activity that fails to achieve this is directly responsible for much of the pollution that leads to environmental and health deficits and may cause major industrial accidents with severe health consequences. Public opinion and consumer demand has supported a marked change in industrial activity, following increased public exposure to health risks and critical review. Small changes in the way that industry does business can unlock money which will not only improve health but also increase profitability. Health is a domain worthy of investment, and healthy products can lead to better business.

Many industries are expanding their view of who has a legitimate stake in their operations. Companies' stakeholders include not only shareholders, lenders and regulators but also employees, customers, suppliers, trade associations, community and environmental groups, the public at large and, in the widest sense, future generations. Industry is increasingly setting public goals for health improvement and pollution reduction and adopting the requisite investment programmes.

POLICY OPTIONS

- Pricing products to reflect the health costs of their production.
- Cleaner processes and preventive strategies, with additional savings in materials, waste disposal costs, and liability charges.
- Establishing and making publicly available inventories of toxic releases.
- Producers marketing products representing a direct risk to health, such as the tobacco industry (as an extreme case), should take full responsibility for the economic and health cost of their products.
- Products barred from use in the country of production should not be exported to other countries; in particular, medical and pharmaceutical products should be regulated by international agreements to ensure safety, environmental soundness and relevance.
- "Healthy company or enterprise" initiatives should be launched to facilitate the exchange of best practice in the workplace, foster partnerships between the private and public sectors, and give firms the opportunity to be "certified" as healthy producers.

RECYCLING WASTE AND IMPROVING HEALTH

In the town of Kalundborg in Denmark, industrial waste and waste process heat are exchanged in a co-operative arrangement among a power plant, an oil refinery, a pharmaceutical manufacturer, a plasterboard factory, a cement producer, farmers and the utility that provides heat for local residents. The arrangement is financially beneficial to all parties and is a working model of a small industrial ecosystem.

Pollution prevention of this type follows a natural hierarchy of waste management options. Waste is reduced at the source. Waste that is produced is reused or recycled, preferably on site and goes directly back into the production process. Waste that cannot be prevented or recycled is treated with the latest technology to detoxify, remove or destroy it.

Source: World Resources Institute. *World resources 1994–95. A guide to the global environment.* Oxford, Oxford University Press, 1994.

Agriculture and food sectors

The agriculture sector provides an essential service to society, producing food, a prerequisite for both health and wellbeing. However, the agricultural sector also has a responsibility to protect and improve the environment, conserve freshwater resources, maintain sustainable development in rural communities, preserve food safety, and contribute to the promotion of good nutrition. Attitudes towards agriculture have recently changed, as consumer criticism of its environmental impact and food safety has increased (e.g. in the development of BSE).

Some 30% of energy consumption in industrialized countries is attributable to the agriculture and food sector. Ten per cent of the energy involved is used in agriculture and livestock production, whereas transport, packaging and preparation of food account for 90%. The potential health benefits of increased food availability need to be balanced against the health impact of long-term climate change. All stakeholders in the agriculture sector have an interest in sustainable food production, protection of the environment and the promotion of health. Stakeholders include primary producers, the agrochemical industry, consumers, and the transport and water abstraction sectors.

POLICY OPTIONS

- Promotion of innovative methods of farming, including setting standards for the agrochemical content of water, land planning, and land use near groundwater abstraction plants and recreational areas.

- Cooperative action at the local level to manage the quality and quantity of freshwater resources.

- Information and legislation to shield ecosystems and consumers from the potential side-effects of genetic manipulation.

- Policies relating to pricing and to research and development, in order to ensure a lower consumption of fats and a higher consumption of vegetables and fruit, particularly targeting poorer socioeconomic groups.

- Increased dialogue with consumers.

- Increased investment in ecologically based agriculture and the production of local safe and sustainable food, to protect livelihoods and health in local communities.

- Close collaboration between WHO, WTO and the Food and Agricultural Organization (FAO), and adherence to the Codex Alimentarius to reduce foodborne diseases transmitted via traded products.

- Assessment of global policies (such as reforms of the EU's common agricultural policy) for their health and environmental impact.

Tourism

Tourism has become one of the important economic sectors in the Region and will become increasingly so in its eastern part. Tourism represented about 5.5% of GDP in the EU in 1990 and is expected to reach a level of nearly 400 million arrivals in European countries by the year 2000. Visitors to cities and heritage sites are expected to increase in the future, as city-based tourism travel becomes more popular. Tourism, which depends for its success on the quality of the natural and built environment, can itself have a negative impact on the environment and so jeopardize its own development. The effects of tourism on the environment include the defacing of landscapes by tourist developments, erosion of coastlines and mountain slopes, accumulation of litter, loss of natural habitats and over-abstraction of water.

Certain areas around the Mediterranean Sea are vulnerable to water shortages during the summer season, when there is an influx of tourists. Contamination of bathing areas with sewage and industrial pollution is widespread throughout all the seas and lakes of the Region. About 70% of municipal sewerage in the Mediterranean region is discharged untreated, and bathing waters and local shellfish are subject to microbial contamination. Accidents, such as drowning and spinal injury, may be associated with recreational use of the water environment, particularly when people are intoxicated. Increased exposure to ultraviolet light through sunbathing can increase the incidence of skin cancer. In mountain areas, the cumulative environmental impacts from skiing are considerable, with the worst effects being seen in the Alps. Each year this area, of approximately 190 000 km^2 receives 100 million tourists. Protection of the environment and protection of tourists and the local population should be the overriding objectives of a sustainable tourist policy.

POLICY OPTIONS

- Investment in infrastructure for water supply, sanitation and waste disposal, and strict regulations relating to industrial and community waste, to preserve tourist and recreational areas and protect tourists.

- Leisure and recreational programmes that promote physical activity, personal development, coping skills and relaxation.

- Accommodation and facilities that promote sexual health, freedom from tobacco smoke, and responsible use of alcohol.

- Measures to ensure a better seasonal spread of tourists.

- Investment in wild habitats and restoration of wild habitats to improve biological diversity.

Finance

The finance sector has an important role to play in supporting work towards environment and health objectives. Pricing and taxation policies are among the strongest means of action for governments, sectors, communities, individuals and society. Yet these instruments are under-utilized when it comes to promoting human development and sustainable economic activity that generate wellbeing and health.

Policy options

- Adoption of fiscal policy to reduce income inequalities, promote sustainable development, protect the environment and promote health.

- Banks to add health impact assessment to the criteria for decisions on loans and investment.

- Government incentives for the production of health-promoting products, and taxes to discourage production of those that damage health.

- Industry pricing policies to include any cost of health damage caused by products.

- Adjustments to the measure of gross national product to reflect positive and negative impacts on human development, health and the environment.

HEALTH SUPPORTIVE TAX REFORM IN THE NETHERLANDS

The 1996 regulatory tax on energy levied taxes on the small-scale use of gas and electricity and certain oil products as a carbon tax, to help achieve the national goals set for CO_2 levels in the year 2000. The US $1 billion revenue is recycled back to households through changes in personal tax income and to business through a reduction of social premiums paid by employers, thus switching taxes from income to taxes on pollutants. Such taxes help to reduce pollution and reflect its true cost for society, leading in the long run to better health from improved air quality, more efficient use of resources, and more sustainable economic performance. The potentially regressive nature of carbon taxes can be balanced by other progressive taxes in the overall tax system.

Source: Vos, H. Environmental taxation in the Netherlands. *In*: O'Riordan, T., ed. *Ecotaxation*. London, Earthscan Publications, 1997.

Social welfare and services

The social sector responds to problems arising from poverty and social exclusion and aims to prevent social ills. As such, the sector has an important contribution to make to the promotion of health and wellbeing. Social welfare policy is under debate in many countries, in the light of a perceived increasing welfare burden resulting from changing demographic trends and persistent unemployment.

Policy options

- Providing a social safety net, especially in economies in transition or decline.

- Ensuring welfare policies that are family-friendly, with caring and parenting given recognition as social rights.

- Balancing parents' need for work and their need to be involved in child care.

- Setting standards for housing, income and social support services tailored to the needs of different target groups.
- Closer collaboration with the health care sector in provision of community-oriented PHC.

The judiciary and legislation

The judiciary has a responsibility for the implementation of legislation to protect the environment and promote health, as well as a responsibility for legal action when environmental and health protection laws are infringed. Globalization has increased the opportunities for avoiding or not complying with regulations in individual countries.

POLICY OPTIONS

- Establishing legislation at national level to facilitate implementation of the World Health Declaration, in partnership with the public health and environment communities.
- Harmonizing legal systems and liability regimes in different countries and ensuring that activities undertaken in one country will not damage the environment or cause injury in others.
- Facilitating litigation against trade and industry in the case of actual health damage.

The media

The mass media in all their forms are increasingly influencing values and shaping public opinion, perceptions and behaviours about health. Mass media influence has been enhanced by rapid developments in communications technology, including telecommunications.

Health and wellness topics are one of the growth areas in media and communications. On the one hand, this gives an opportunity to provide health information and publicly expose activities that lead to health risk. On the other hand, there is danger that advertising and marketing in all its forms serves the interests of risk producers, for example the alcohol and tobacco industries, in promoting unhealthy choices.

POLICY OPTIONS

- Healthy communication partnerships (involving governments, county and municipal authorities, health institutes, industry and trade, consumer organizations) to provide accurate, relevant and rapid information about health.
- Training and ethical codes for all health communicators.

The health sector

This chapter does not cover the health sector, although it is an important motivator for, and partner in, multisectoral action for health. The joint responsibility and partnership of sectors is taken up in Chapter 7, whereas Chapter 6 focuses on action inside the health sector.

Chapter 6

An outcome-oriented health sector

> Target 15 – An integrated health sector
> Target 16 – Managing for quality of care
> Target 17 – Funding health services and allocating resources
> Target 18 – Developing human resources for health

6.1 Introduction

This HFA strategy necessarily takes a broad perspective on the breadth and content of the health sector – inevitably, as so many of the determinants of health lie outside the purview and influence of clinical care. The health sector, under the governance of a ministry or department of health, has the primary objective of health improvement: it delivers health services, is responsible for health policy and management, and carries out activities oriented to both the individual citizen/patient and the community/population.

Health services include those structures and personnel that work for health promotion, disease prevention, treatment and rehabilitation, using resources specifically identified and allocated for these purposes.

Health services make a highly significant contribution to population health. They use a considerable amount of economic resources and count among each country's major employers. They also foster a feeling of security in individuals and a climate of confidence in society; factors which are important for the development of the economy and, more generally, for society as a whole.

The conditions within society in which health services are delivered are undergoing a substantial demographic, economic, political and social transformation, and demand pressures are increasing.

The rise in the numbers of the elderly and increasing levels of poverty, unemployment and migration (all of which are associated with higher levels of chronic disease and disability) are exerting an upward pressure on overall health services; and new and expensive technologies and treatments are also major contributory factors to cost increases. This has given rise to cost concerns in all countries.

LJUBLJANA CHARTER

The Ljubljana Conference on Health Care Reforms was a cornerstone in terms of analysing the trends in reforming health care in Europe, identifying the challenges and constraints, and being a catalyst for sharing experience. The whole process also led to an exploration of the shared principles underlying health care systems. As a result of these efforts, the Ljubljana Charter was adopted by all Member States in 1996.

The Charter addresses health care reforms in the specific context of the European Region and is centred on the principle that health care should first and foremost lead to better health and quality of life for people. It emphasizes the fact that health care reforms should be an integral part of an overall health policy. The first step is to develop an HFA policy, and then to develop appropriate reform strategies. The Charter also emphasizes that health care systems need to:

- be governed by the principles of human dignity, equity, solidarity and professional ethics
- relate to clear targets for health gain
- address citizens' needs
- aim at continuous improvements in the quality of care
- ensure financing that will enable health care to be provided to all citizens in a sustainable way
- be oriented towards primary health care.

The Charter highlights the principles for managing change effectively: developing coherent health care policies, listening to the citizen's voice and choice, reshaping health care delivery, reorienting human resources, strengthening management and learning from experience.

The Ljubljana Charter has significant implications for health care reform in the European context. In the past decade, health care reform focused on other issues rather than on health. The main concerns were to ensure a market orientation and cost-containment, and many tools were developed to create a competitive market in health care. The process of the Ljubljana Conference and development of the Charter questioned these reform tools, especially the competition-oriented ones, in terms of their impact on health. This showed that financial mechanisms and leverage systems need to focus on the supply side, rather than on the demand side, in order to improve health outcomes. The Ljubljana Charter has succeeded in drawing attention back to health gain and in providing an outcome-oriented policy direction.

Source: Ljubljana Charter on reforming health care in Europe. Copenhagen, WHO Regional Office for Europe, 1996 (document EUR/ICP/CARE 9401/CN01 Rev.1).

In recent years, many health care reforms have taken place throughout the Region. Many governments have reconsidered their role in the provision of health services and started to introduce various market mechanisms into service delivery. The purchaser/provider split, the introduction of competitive elements into health services, and various payment mechanisms, are just some of the approaches adopted. Although the policy intentions in many countries include reorienting health care systems towards PHC, these intentions have often not been reflected in practice. More attention has, however, been paid to the introduction, training and functions of general practitioners/family physicians.

The gap in health service provision between countries, and between regions and social groups within countries, is widening, and for many countries in the eastern part of the Region the situation is now critical. Often the accessibility and quality of health services have suffered. Generally, an over-emphasis on care itself, particularly curative care, continues to dominate, while health promotion, disease prevention and rehabilitation efforts receive far less attention than they should.

Until now, the prevailing international model has been to see clinical patient care and "public health" as two separate entities, with different orientations, resource allocation principles and management. Furthermore, within clinical care itself the hospital and primary care levels have far too often had little interaction – or even been antagonists, fighting among themselves for status, influence and resources.

The HFA approach offers a new perspective, one that focuses attention on the final health outcome and sees health promotion/disease prevention/diagnosis/treatment/rehabilitation/care, not as separate entities, but as one continuous link of actions to improve health gain. However, to turn this general statement into a reality requires:

- a common denominator to compare the relative effectiveness of each of the above elements; this can only be a measured improvement in the health status of the target population;
- a management system which ensures that the different elements in the system are resourced according to their relative value, that they operate so as to optimize their individual and combined actions, and that they are monitored/evaluated on the basis of their impact on agreed health outcome indicators.

Thus, embracing the HFA perspective means adopting a common yardstick and ensuring closer cooperation between patient care and public health. Increasingly, such an approach will support the concept of public health management through broad condition-specific programmes of care in which health promotion, disease prevention, therapy and rehabilitation are considered together and where judgements about the choice and balance of services to be provided are made on the basis of evidence.

6.2 Integrating primary health care and hospital services

Such an approach will need to be supported by a health service and care system that is structurally and functionally more integrated, whereas at present health services are often fragmented, both horizontally and vertically. Care is often episodic and split up among several medical specialists, nurses and other health professionals, rather than being organized around the concept of a multi-professional team providing comprehensive and horizontally integrated care. The vertical integration between primary, secondary and tertiary care is also often weak, and continuity of care between the various levels not ensured in many countries.

Different approaches to the organization and provision of PHC have been followed in different countries, including polyclinics, group practices, and single-handed practice. In many countries, health care is uncoordinated and responsibility is divided between different authorities. Parallel vertical care structures still exist in several Member States, for TB, STDs, and maternal and child health, for instance, performing functions that could and should be provided in a coordinated and integrated way.

Environmental health services are often not well integrated with other health services. In some countries, PHC has been used as a way of introducing private practice into the health care system, without due regard for how equity, accessibility and continuity of services should be safeguarded.

The full potential of PHC to reduce the numerous unnecessary admissions to hospital has certainly not been realised. In many countries, hospitals continue to dominate health care, often treating patients who could and should be better treated at the community level. Although in theory they can offer facilities not only for the rapid admission of patients from PHC but also for their return to that level, this often does not happen properly in practice.

The role of people in caring for themselves and determining their own health is not sufficiently recognized, and the local community is not involved enough in dealing with problems of health and health care. Recent trends have increased the potential role of citizens in health care; they are more informed thanks to better education, the mass media and computer technology, all of which have made information more accessible. There is increased scope for self-medication as access to appropriate information is provided and safety concerns are ruled out.

Hospital services underwent considerable expansion in the European Region during the 1960s, 1970s and the beginning of the 1980s but have since experienced increasing difficulties. In western Europe, years of cost-cutting have in many countries led to a substantial decrease in the number of hospital beds and strong pressure for higher productivity. An intensive pace of working, increasing stress levels and decreasing continuity of care has been the resulting picture in many hospitals.

In the more eastern parts of the Region, the very large number of hospital beds (a legacy of health care policy in the past), combined with a severe economic crisis during the 1990s has created an extremely difficult situation characterized by dilapidated buildings, worn-out equipment, lack of basic supplies and a financial inability to profit from new breakthroughs in hospital technology.

> **TARGET 15 – AN INTEGRATED HEALTH SECTOR**
>
> BY THE YEAR 2010, PEOPLE IN THE REGION SHOULD HAVE MUCH BETTER ACCESS TO FAMILY- AND COMMUNITY-ORIENTED PRIMARY HEALTH CARE, SUPPORTED BY A FLEXIBLE AND RESPONSIVE HOSPITAL SYSTEM.
>
> In particular:
>
> 15.1 at least 90% of countries should have comprehensive primary health care services, ensuring continuity of care through efficient and cost-effective systems of referral to, and feedback from, secondary and tertiary hospital services;
>
> 15.2 at least 90% of countries should have family health physicians and nurses working at the core of this integrated primary health care service, using multiprofessional teams from the health, social and other sectors and involving local communities;
>
> 15.3 at least 90% of countries should have health services that ensure individuals' participation and recognizes and supports people as producers of health care.

PROPOSED STRATEGIES

Both for western and for eastern Europe, the only sensible way out of the present quandary is to ensure a more integrated health service system where PHC is equipped to solve all problems that can be effectively dealt with at that level, while hospital care is reserved for those that cannot. This approach emphasizes the essential priority to be given to PHC and aims at utilizing the resources of society in such a way as to secure the maximum health outcomes. Such a system promotes integrated primary, secondary and tertiary health care and will be economically, politically and socially suited to the unique conditions of the society in which the care is provided.

6.2.1 Functions of integrated health services

Needs assessment

The functions of a health service should meet the needs of the society, with an assessment of those needs, using applied epidemiological methodology, taken as a basis for service planning and provision. The special needs of children, the elderly, marginalized social groups and, indeed, the whole population served (in view of the increasing number of homeless and otherwise "excluded" people in all countries) should be addressed in this manner.

Priorities for programmes and activities thus identified may relate to various functions of health services, such as health promotion and disease prevention, or to problems outside the usual remit of the health services, such as those related to the environment and social conditions in the community.

Health promotion and disease prevention

Health services extend beyond diagnosis and treatment – through health promotion and disease prevention, they contribute to health throughout the life cycle. These services should perceive human beings holistically and aim at their overall physical, mental and social wellbeing. They can most easily be integrated and provided within PHC.

Health promotion advice on important lifestyle issues such as nutrition, exercise, consumption of alcohol and cessation of smoking is most effective if it is persistent, consistent and continuous, and if it is offered to families and communities at all levels. Within this population context, individual advice can be given on an opportunistic basis to those who attend health services for whatever reason. Appropriate screening activities to detect preconditions for, or early stages of, disease must be systematically organized at PHC level, as must the necessary vaccination services.

SMOKING CESSATION INTERVENTIONS IN PRIMARY CARE

In the United Kingdom, integration of the national health targets within the regulatory system has led to local purchasing plans addressing the national targets, along with locally identified health priorities. In addition, general practitioners' contracts have a specific requirement that they must give health promotion advice to patients. The purchasing of health promotion services through contracts has led to the evaluation of health promotion interventions in both clinical and cost–effectiveness terms. It has been shown that in smoking cessation, interventions provided at the primary care level such as brief advice and counselling are very cost-effective in producing population health gains.

Sources: European health care reform. Copenhagen, WHO Regional Office for Europe, 1997 (WHO Regional Publications, European Series, No. 72); Buck, D. The cost–effectiveness of smoking cessation interventions: what do we know? *International journal of health education*, **35**(2): 44–52 (1997).

The role of PHC in meeting environmental health needs should be reassessed. The countries in the western part of the Region may need better links and organizational support for this role, whereas in the eastern part better integration is needed, especially through sanitary/epidemiological services in the NIS.

Diagnosis and treatment

Timely diagnosis and effective treatment of diseases must be ensured. The former will require both the general population and health professionals to be knowledgeable about the diseases that they will encounter at various stages of the life cycle, as well as their symptoms. Health professionals should be well trained so that they can explore, during consultations, the possible diseases correlating to the age span of the patient.

The pattern of fragmented care for single episodes of illness, often by different medical specialists, should be superseded by integrated health care, characterized by comprehensiveness and personal continuity, and by a working relationship between care providers and the general population based on mutual trust. Particular attention needs to be paid to emergency services for acute illness, accidents and disasters.

Rehabilitation

Rehabilitation requires continuity, dialogue, follow-up and perseverance. It is also a function of all three levels of care. Special services, such as physiotherapy, speech therapy, and occupational and social rehabilitation services, have specific, vital functions to perform.

The social and welfare services, which are outside the usual scope of health care, have an important role to play in social rehabilitation, as well as in supporting patients with chronic disabilities and in counselling patients who need help in coping with the problems of daily living and survival in today's complex societies. PHC should be the natural focal point for these networks.

6.2.2 Organization of integrated health services

Family-oriented care

As mentioned in Chapter 5, families (households) are the basic unit of society where health care providers will be able not only to address patients' somatic physical complaints but also to take into account the psychological and social aspects of their condition. It is important for PHC providers to know the circumstances in which patients live: their housing, family circumstances, work, and social or physical environment may all have a considerable bearing on their illness. Unless care providers are aware of these circumstances, presenting symptoms may be misinterpreted and conditions may go unrecognized and untreated. The result may be unnecessary diagnostic and treatment procedures, thus increasing costs without helping to address the real problems.

Serving a specified population improves the relationship between health professionals and the population. One feature that contributes strongly to providing the full range of services described so far is that each family health physician and family health nurse should serve a specified population, defined either as a geographical catchment area or through enrolment on a list. In both cases, it is also important for people to be able to choose freely a professional whom they can identify as "their own" from among the list of professionals practising in the area. The establishment of such a link between health professionals and the population makes it very much easier to carry out PHC functions and activities. It also ensures effectiveness, since physicians can more easily and quickly recognize the health problems of the particular patients they know throughout their life course. Furthermore, continuity of care is ensured as one person is followed by the same health professional for a continuous period.

Self-care

As mentioned in section 4.4, much more health can be created if health care systems recognize and acknowledge the actual and potential contribution people can make to their own health (self-care) and take active steps to empower them to do so. It is a public responsibility to ensure that citizens receive extensive, accurate and timely information on health and health care through various communication channels; information itself exerts a key influence on people's health and on how they use health care services.

Health professionals should also act as agents, guides and counsellors for their patients in their relationships with other agencies and with social and other health-related services. Both at national and at local community levels, the creation of patients' organizations should be encouraged and their actions supported.

> **PORTUGUESE PHARMACIES PROVIDE COUNSELLING SERVICES TO THE COMMUNITY**
>
> One of the counselling services is a needle exchange programme, "*Say no to a used needle*", to help prevent sexual and blood transmission of HIV among drug users. The project has been running since October 1993 through the 2500 pharmacies spread across the country, and it has been a success as measured by the number of used syringes and acceptance of the project by drug users. Another counselling service is helping to prevent primary and secondary diabetes, by promoting early diagnosis and by advising people about healthy lifestyles – advice that is taken up by a number of "patients". The European Forum of Pharmaceutical Associations and the WHO Regional Office for Europe (EuroPharm Forum) promotes similar projects in a number of countries.
>
> *Source*: Matias, L. & Teles, A. Portuguese National Pharmaceutical Association (unpublished data). Soares, M.A. et al. Lisbon, Santa Maria Hospital (unpublished data).

In many countries, there is a growing vogue for the use of "alternative" treatments and service providers. The perception of human beings as holistic entities with the right to make free choices recognizes and tolerates, even welcomes, the existence of alternative health care alongside conventional medicine. However, in this area, too, high ethical standards need to be met, consumers must be protected against exploitation, and public funds should be used only for treatments with scientifically proved effect.

Home care

The need for home care is increasing in line with the changing demographic structure, improvements in technology and the demands of the population. The home is the setting where health care is most commonly provided. Regular home visits by health personnel play an important role in health promotion and disease prevention services. Follow-up of chronically ill or convalescing patients generally takes place in the home environment.

PHC services should take on a special role in this respect towards their population, acting together with them as co-producers of health and health care: informing and advising people on how to preserve their health and supporting them, with care provided at home, when they care for themselves.

Primary care must also support physically disabled people or those with mental health problems, making major efforts to provide the care that will keep them functioning in their home environment and, if possible, in the labour market. However, sheltered accommodation must be provided for those who need it – only in severe cases should resort be made to nursing-home care. Health programmes for these client groups must be established jointly by the health services, social services, schools, NGOs and, in particular, self-help groups.

Lastly, PHC must also support the elderly, in view of their growing numbers and increasing social isolation and hardship, especially among those suffering from chronic disease and disability. It should provide and coordinate care for this group of patients, including home care and – when required – institutional care in nursing homes. These need to be designed to cater for the varying needs of different patients: facilities for day care, night care and short- and long-term care should be part of, or at least work closely with, PHC teams.

Schools and workplaces

As mentioned in Chapter 5, schools and workplaces require more attention as important settings for the provision of PHC. School health services have important promotive, preventive, diagnostic and therapeutic roles to play concerning children's health and educational attainment.

Occupational health services are concerned with all aspects of the relationship between occupation and health. Workplaces require special attention in terms of preventive services and work safety. While they usually require a separate organizational structure, they are none the less part of PHC and should work in close liaison with other primary care settings.

Referral systems

An effective referral system requires a well organized referral and feedback mechanism between primary, secondary and tertiary care. Not all the conditions that patients present can be dealt with by PHC. Patients who have complicated or life-threatening conditions must be referred as required to the appropriate specialist in good time, in order to avoid unnecessary complications and unwarranted disability. The ability to recognize those situations that require referral is one of the important skills that all health professionals working in PHC should develop. A necessary corollary of referral is the two-way exchange of information between primary, secondary and tertiary levels, in order to ensure follow-up and continuity of care, since PHC services will have the responsibility of monitoring and assisting patients after the care given at the secondary and tertiary levels. Many Member States have gone further, making it mandatory that the patient's first consultation with the health services should be in a PHC setting, which is thus formally identified as the "gatekeeper". Indeed, such a system contributes to efficiency, since unnecessary or overly intrusive consultations with secondary and tertiary care services are avoided. Establishing a gatekeeping system certainly requires well trained physicians working in well organized PHC settings. It should be noted that patients may be referred not only to secondary and tertiary medical services but also to other health professionals working at the primary level, or to agencies outside the health sector such as social welfare services.

6.2.3 Primary health care facilities

PHC facilities can ensure networking among the various settings in which health services and other sectors operate. Facilities such as group practices, polyclinics, health centres and any site that provides first-contact care play a crucial role in carrying out the main functions of PHC, bringing together multidisciplinary health care teams of professionals, local institutions, NGOs, local schools, the local media and companies, for example, and applying a multisectoral approach to the problems that need to be addressed.

6.2.4 Hospitals

Secondary and tertiary care support PHC by providing technologically-based diagnosis, treatment and rehabilitation. In most Member States, secondary and tertiary care should more clearly serve and support primary care, concentrating on those functions that cannot be performed effectively by the latter. Patients who can be served in a clinically sound way in a PHC setting should be.

Planning secondary and tertiary care facilities in accordance with the principle of a population-based "regionalized" system allows for more rational use of expensive technologies and of the expertise of highly trained personnel. In this respect, regional health administrators and hospital management personnel need to have much better information about the health needs of the population they serve, in order to plan a rational hierarchy of services and to assess whether health problems are being adequately dealt with or not. This will require better information and management systems to cover both patient care and administrative procedures.

In order to rationalize the use of secondary and tertiary health care settings, "substitution policies" must be introduced for referrals – this will entail changing the locality for diagnosis and treatment to take in other facilities in addition to conventional hospital services, and transferring responsibilities and tasks between health personnel. A common theme has been the reduction in the number of patients who need to stay in hospital overnight. "Day care hospitals", "short stay hospitals" and "hospitals without beds" describe services which provide much shorter-term, ambulatory care. The term "hospital at home" has been used to describe very special outreach services organized by hospitals (for example, for chronic patients on home haemodialysis). In the eastern part of the Region, the high number of hospital beds needs to be reduced; however, this reduction should be made in parallel with the introduction of substitution policies.

Hospitals in the European Region now often serve both acute and chronic patients, but these two categories need to be better differentiated in order to optimize the use of resources and staff expertise. Acute hospitals should provide acute care in more serious cases needing access to their clinical facilities for diagnosis, treatment and rehabilitation. By contrast, long-stay institutions for the chronically ill and other extended care establishments should try to ensure a more home-like environment and the care appropriate to the special needs of their residents. Such institutions should not be too large and are best seen as part of PHC, or of the social sector, rather than of the hospital sector.

Besides staffing costs, hospitals' running costs are being driven up by the costs of maintaining their infrastructure, while safety of equipment, waste management plant and other physical and technical features require constant upgrading. This is another reason for substituting the most cost-effective PHC alternatives for the use of these expensive facilities, when it is clinically sound to do so.

6.3 Managing for quality in health outcomes

Health development is intended to contribute to health improvement, and systematic measurement of health outcomes for the Region as a whole and for each Member State has taken place since 1984, using outcome-oriented HFA indicators tailored to each regional HFA target. However, only some countries have set their own specific targets and indicators, and far too few use health outcomes as the main parameter for managing the health sector. In fewer countries still are health outcomes used as the main parameter for managing individual health service institutions. No country, either in the European Region or elsewhere, has a system where all clinicians receive continuous feedback on the results of their own patient care.

This situation reveals a very serious flaw in health care management philosophy and practice. This flaw prevents the health system from being properly focused and leads to much current practice in the European Region being below the assumed quality; it is also wasteful of its resources. The major challenge in health care for all Member States in the European Region is therefore to refocus the management of health services and care towards measuring the true impact of different interventions on the health of the population; the use of health outcome indicators offers a unifying concept for doing this.

Until recently, it was generally assumed that well trained physicians and other health care providers, who had systematic information about scientific innovations and who were working in well equipped health care institutions, would automatically produce homogenous and high-quality health care. However, a steadily mounting body of evidence shows that this is not the case and that, in spite of existing knowledge, there are wide (and sometimes very large) variations in the outcomes of care. Such differences in outcome are found not only between countries or regions within countries, but also between institutions, hospital departments and individual health care providers.

Information systems at all levels should clearly support informed management and continuous quality development. However, in the European Region, almost all individual health service institutions and providers currently lack basic information about the quality of the care they provide in their daily practice. The situation is much better with regard to population-based information, since the (over 200) regional HFA indicators agreed on by Member States since 1984 have enabled a unique database to be built up for comparing different health strategies.

TARGET 16 – MANAGING FOR QUALITY OF CARE

BY THE YEAR 2010, MEMBER STATES SHOULD ENSURE THAT THE MANAGEMENT OF THE HEALTH SECTOR, FROM POPULATION-BASED HEALTH PROGRAMMES TO INDIVIDUAL PATIENT CARE AT THE CLINICAL LEVEL, IS ORIENTED TOWARDS HEALTH OUTCOMES.

In particular:

16.1 the effectiveness of major public health strategies should be assessed in terms of health outcomes, and decisions regarding alternative strategies for dealing with individual health problems should increasingly be taken by comparing health outcomes and their cost–effectiveness;

16.2 all countries should have a nationwide mechanism for continuous monitoring and development of the quality of care for at least ten major health conditions, including measurement of health impact, cost–effectiveness and patient satisfaction;

16.3 health outcomes in at least five of the above health conditions should show a significant improvement, and surveys should show an increase in patient's satisfaction with the quality of services received and heightened respect for their rights.

PROPOSED STRATEGIES

Quality means degree of excellence, and quality development should not be seen as an administrative control to ensure the attainment of a predetermined quality level – rather, it is a dynamic process that encourages a continuous, innovative improvement in health care outcome. It is therefore essential that health services should be organized in such a way that health outcome will be the main concern in identifying inputs, defining processes and evaluating outputs. The whole process should target health improvement, patient satisfaction and cost–effectiveness, as opposed to traditional management practices in which the system has been viewed from an input perspective, with plans developed according to inputs.

National and professional policies

A first requirement is to develop a common policy for a country that adheres to these principles, and WHO's Regional Office for Europe has worked with national administrations and professional organizations to develop such models (see below).

> **NATIONAL POLICIES FOR CONTINUOUS QUALITY OF CARE DEVELOPMENT**
>
> Continuous quality of care development has been taken up by several countries on the basis of national policies on the quality of care. Such policies have been developed with WHO assistance in Denmark (1993), Belgium (1995), Slovenia and Poland, and are under implementation and/or development in, Hungary and Lithuania, among others. In Denmark, formulation of the policy has been followed with the establishment of numerous new databases and development of evidence-based quality criteria. The European Forum of National Medical Associations (NMAs) and WHO have developed and endorsed a model quality of care development policy for NMAs which is in accordance with national policies and are promoting their development among its members.
>
> *Sources*: Blomhøj, G. et al. *Continuous quality development: a proposed national policy*. Copenhagen, WHO Regional Office for Europe, 1995 (document EUR/ICP/CLR 059); Borgions, J. et al. *Développement continu de la qualité des soins: Proposition de politique nationale*. Brussels, Ministère de la santé publique et de l'environnement, and Copenhagen, WHO Regional Office for Europe, 1995; Recommendations for national medical associations regarding quality of care development. *Medisch Contact*, 38: 166 (1993).

Outcome indicators

A basic minimum of relevant and measurable outcome indicators – particularly health outcome indicators – need to be developed to support the whole range of action between public health work and individual clinical care, and they should be internationally agreed on (so as to learn from international comparisons), regularly monitored and evaluated as part of the health services' routine operations. For any health programme such outcome indicators, scientifically valid and based on practical experience, should cover the various aspects of health care (health promotion, disease prevention, treatment and rehabilitation) and be used to compare the relative value of each when planning and managing such programmes.

Outcome indicators help to measure which interventions are effective, and they should be used for monitoring daily patient care and for assessing new diagnostic and therapeutic technologies (including new pharmaceutical products and medical equipment), during both initial trials and subsequent routine use. They can also become an important tool in new management techniques, such as monitoring the implementation of contracts between purchasers and providers of health services and care. This has implication for the work of public health management experts (see section 6.5 below).

Continuous quality development using documented outcome measurement and evidence-based medicine contributes to more effective application of diagnostic and curative interventions and to a reduction of unnecessary expenditure on procedures and pharmaceuticals.

The education and training of health professionals must equip them with the skills required to be active participants in this process, providing them with the means to assess the quality and outcome of their clinical work as a necessary step in improving health care delivery.

Evidence-based care

Quality is assessed on the basis of evidence and achievement of the best results is identified using scientific knowledge. Interventions (whether in the health services or in health care itself) must always be based on scientifically validated evidence. Efforts to systematically sample such evidence for different interventions and to ensure its acceptance by health care providers are therefore an important concern.

In this context, reviewing and synthesizing the results of research, maintaining registers and databases based on agreed outcome indicators, and disseminating findings to decision-makers and to providers and users of services are important functions. These findings can be seen as providing "benchmarks" of best practice for others to match or surpass.

Guidelines for clinical practice should be developed on the basis of best measured outcomes; they should be "owned" by those who will use them, and they should be frequently updated in order not to lead to stagnation. A dynamic search for better ways forward must come both from basic research and from innovations in daily practice.

> **TARGETED PROGRAMMES BASED ON SOUND DATA LEAD TO SUSTAINABLE HEALTH IMPROVEMENTS**
>
> In Stockholm, Sweden, a programme for detection and treatment of diabetes retinopathy in line with the objectives of the St Vincent Declaration has shown remarkable results: during a period of ten years, the blindness rates in this region were reduced by 60%. It is suggested that this programme can be as successful in many more regions, since the project demonstrates that an improvement has been made even in a country which has already a good and modern health care delivery system.
>
> Such programmes have to be developed on sound clinical data. The Norwegian hip register, which is run by the Norwegian Orthopedic Society, has led to a continuous registration of all surgical procedures related to the implantation and later revision surgery of all hip prothesis. The data are fed back in anonymized form to all participating centres. This leads to a much more focused approach in the development and provision of hip surgery in Norway, as discussions are based on "real data". For instance, the database has contributed strongly to the streamlining of medical procedures in hip surgery, thus providing better quality of care.
>
> *Sources*: Stæhr Johansen, K. et al. Improving health of people with diabetes: The "End of the beginning". *Diabetes nutrition and metabolism*, **10**(3): (1997); Bäcklund, L.B. et al. New blindness in diabetes reduced by more than one-third in Stockholm county. *Diabetic medicine*, **14**: 732–740 (1997); L.I. Havelin, Chairman, Norwegian Hip Register, personal communication, 1998.

Information systems

A major strategy for quality development is to establish an information system at the clinical level, providing feedback to individual health professionals on the outcomes of the care they deliver. (See also 7.2.2.) An information system of this kind should be designed to allow the individual providers to compare each others' outcomes on an anonymous basis (as otherwise information given will tend to be less correct and the system resisted); experience has shown that this can have an immediate and major positive effect on the quality of care provided by individual health professionals who, when they realize that their performance and use of technology may not be optimal, have a major ethical incentive to change.

Such systems also provide a unique opportunity to identify those who really are the best achievers in terms of health care outcomes. Surprisingly, they are not always those thought to be the best, but instead may be more innovative, more concerned with their patients or more thorough in their work. This changes the whole concept from one of quality assurance to quality development, whereby the results of the best achievers constantly "pull" the rest of the field forward. This approach opens up the search for new ideas and turns the quest for better quality into a continuous and dynamic process, where superior performance can quickly be recognized.

Based on information on quality compiled in aggregate at population levels (e.g. the local community, the county or region, or the country as a whole), quality improvement targets should be set for a given period and quality indicators agreed upon.

Patient satisfaction

Citizens may be empowered by providing the necessary information to enable them to participate in evaluating the quality of care. Community participation in decision-making for health care should be ensured at all levels. Many self-help groups and patients' organizations have been set up (associations of patients with chronic renal failure, haemophilia, thalassaemia, diabetes and asthma, and associations of relatives of patients suffering from mental disorders, for instance) and they play a very valuable role as advocates of improvement in the services provided. They make a noteworthy contribution to monitoring the quality of services and to improving the management of the condition concerned; this parallels and sometimes overlaps with the outcomes and quality movement within the health sector itself.

Like health care providers and purchasers, the public need good information, in particular about what they can reasonably expect in terms of quality and outcome of care, in order to make meaningful choices, to have an informed dialogue with health care providers and to decide how to arrange their lives when they are ill or under treatment. One explicit aim of health care systems in the future should be to provide citizens and patients with information, in order to empower them and improve their health.

Many European countries have chosen to adopt special legislation on patients' rights. Another approach is to implement a widely accepted patients' charter. The Declaration on the Promotion of Patients' Rights in Europe (Amsterdam, 1994) provides a useful framework for countries wishing to take action in this area. Possibly the most significant effects of this trend are that patients will understand more about their health condition and treatment, and health care workers will become more respectful of patients' needs and views and be more supportive in helping them to manage their own disease in a better way.

6.3.1 Application of management tools to obtain outcomes

Management flexibility

A greater degree of decentralization in management has much to offer in terms of improving the performance of the health service. Increased autonomy is also compatible with competition; the latter can be encouraged through a greater degree of patient choice and through mechanisms for allocating resources in the light of quality indicators.

Contracting arrangements between purchasers and providers of health care can also be useful tools in this respect. They can enable purchasers to concentrate on identifying the population's health needs and on meeting them through coordinated contracts with a range of service and care providers. Such competition between providers is also compatible with a regionalized system, but only if purchasers have a coherent strategic framework and there is reasonable cooperation between providers. Contracts can also support quality development, if agreed quality indicators are incorporated in the bills that providers submit to third-party payers. In such situations the confidentiality of individual providers must be safeguarded. Aggregates of data at population level will serve as one input for health and health care assessments and for future target-setting and contracting in a context of continuous quality development.

It is, however, health care professionals, not managers, who ultimately decide what is to be done in their daily clinical work with individual patients, so managers must be sensitive to the views of both patients and professionals. Information technology should be harnessed to improve the quality of care and the efficiency of diagnostic and therapeutic departments. Better communication between hospitals and PHC can ensure continuity of care.

6.3.2 Planning inputs for outcomes

Sound planning mechanisms need to be in place that take good outcomes as their fundamental goal. Inputs and processes should be planned in order to ensure health outcome, patient satisfaction and cost–effectiveness. Among these three quality spheres, an explicit choice is made in favour of health outcomes as the most effective tool with which to achieve the other two. An approach designed to foster continuous quality development requires health professionals to be trained as communicators, working towards patient satisfaction, and to be concerned about the cost implications of their interventions.

Human resources should be planned with the appropriate skill mix to ensure the desired outcomes. Their education and training will provide them with the necessary knowledge to perform their tasks, as well as with the skills to measure and evaluate their outcomes.

The allocation of financial resources should reflect the outcomes achieved, and include incentives for improving the quality of care. Selection of the appropriate technology, the provision of pharmaceuticals and the physical infrastructure should be planned accordingly.

6.4 Funding and allocation of resources for health services and care

6.4.1 Financial resources

Level of financing

Adequate financial resources are a prerequisite for the operation of health services and the delivery of care. Health expenditure as a percentage of GNP depends largely on the economic status of a country, and varies from 3.1% to 10.7% across the Region. Clearly, in some countries of the Region the absolute level of public spending on health is simply inadequate to meet anything like the population's reasonable requirements. In many countries, health promotion and disease prevention are inadequately funded. All too often, measures aimed at containing costs have been targeted at patients and users of the health system, rather than at health care institutions and providers.

The trends in the Region indicate the likelihood that additional resources and investments will be directed towards meeting human development needs, especially in health, education and culture. Health care is part of a continuum of investing in health.

Resources can be released if steps are taken to focus attention on the quality of care and on planning and managing the whole health sector, weighing up the relative values of health promotion, disease prevention, diagnosis/treatment, rehabilitation and care. These resources can then be used to fund some of the new investments that will be required to apply more effective (but often expensive) new technologies and to care for increasing numbers of elderly people.

Sources of funding

Sources of funding vary from country to country, ranging from tax-based to insurance-based systems. There is a considerable debate about how best to fund services so as to maintain universal access and financial sustainability. Most often, a mix of these systems is seen. The countries in the eastern part of the Region have largely implemented tax-based systems, although some are in the process of introducing health insurance. Other countries, especially in the south of the Region, are moving from insurance-based systems to tax-based ones.

Private insurance schemes are often operated in a way that corrodes social solidarity through the use of individual risk rating – a particularly pernicious type of cover. In such cases, the basis of payments by an individual to the health insurance company takes the form of risk-adjusted premiums that reflect his or her health status. A system based on competition between private health insurers will violate the principles of equity and solidarity if insurers seek to select good risks.

Allocation of financial resources

Resources should be allocated in the light of a society's needs and priorities. Choices have to be made between geographical areas and services and between particular forms of treatment, and about whether to provide innovative or expensive procedures.

In response to concerns about how best to allocate financial resources to facilities and services so as to maximize health gain and reduce costs, several countries have started to examine priority-setting in a more systematic and explicit way in recent years. Setting priorities involves several levels of decision, ranging from those to do with overall funding of health services in relation to other competing claims for resources, to those related to the treatment of individual patients. A number of countries in the Region have moved from integrated models of service provision towards separating public, or quasi-public, third-party payers from providers.

Geographical allocation of resources mostly does not correspond to need. Especially in the eastern part of the Region, infrastructure-based norms are more likely to encourage excess provision than respond to actual needs.

Provider payments

At present, three different systems are used by countries in the European Region to pay primary care physicians – salary, capitation (i.e. an annual amount per person for whom the physician has permanent responsibility) and fee-for-service. Allowances to reward good practice can be combined with any of these three systems. Each has its advantages and disadvantages, and none of them alone can meet all the policy objectives.

Providers of secondary and tertiary care should be paid to contain costs and ensure value for money in terms of health. Traditional approaches to paying hospitals (based on inputs or intermediate outputs such as beds, rather than on outcomes) are not a convenient means of ensuring that these aims are attained, and retrospective hospital payment systems based on service volume are open-ended, making it difficult to control costs and utilization.

TARGET 17 – FUNDING HEALTH SERVICES AND ALLOCATING RESOURCES

BY THE YEAR 2010, MEMBER STATES SHOULD HAVE SUSTAINABLE FINANCING AND RESOURCE ALLOCATION MECHANISMS FOR HEALTH CARE SYSTEMS BASED ON THE PRINCIPLES OF EQUAL ACCESS, COST–EFFECTIVENESS, SOLIDARITY, AND OPTIMUM QUALITY.

In particular:

17.1 spending on health services should be adequate, while corresponding to the health needs of the population;

17.2 resources should be allocated between health promotion and protection, treatment and care, taking account of health impact, cost–effectiveness and the available scientific evidence;

17.3 funding systems for health care guarantee universal coverage, solidarity and sustainability.

Sustainable funding for health services

The level of financial resources required to operate a health service is impossible to specify in absolute terms, and it is not easy to correlate that level of funding with a country's health experience. Certainly the amount should be affordable by the country and enough to meet the needs of both health promotion and the provision of effective and high quality care. These objectives are simply stated but much more difficult to reconcile in practice. Nevertheless, a comparative analysis of current European experience suggests that 7–10% of GDP may provide for a reasonable spread of health system capacity and performance, dependent of course on an adequate overall level of national GDP. Furthermore, in most countries expenditure trends over time ought to show an increase in the share of resources allocated to health promotion and disease prevention, and to PHC.

It should be noted that this range is indicative only; individual countries must determine the best level based on their economic resources, their health experience, and their need for health promotion and the provision of effective and high-quality care.

Collective funding and solidarity

Regardless of the main method of funding used, governments, as the elected representatives of the people, have the responsibility of ensuring solidarity and universal access to health services, as well as of containing overall costs. Governments may have different positions, for instance as the main source of funds (in countries with taxation-based arrangements) or as the regulator of contributions (in countries with social insurance systems). In both cases, however, their role in ensuring universal access and solidarity is crucial and should not be diminished.

Measures should be taken to promote collective funding, whether by insurance or taxation, to ensure solidarity and "risk pooling". A core concern in countries engaged in transforming their funding systems is to balance the principle of solidarity with increasing pressures to introduce competition mechanisms, which are considered to promote quality of care and efficient use of resources. In terms of solidarity, sizeable out-of-pocket payments at the point of use are the most regressive form of payment for health care, since they represent a greater share of income for the poor who are also higher consumers of care. Collective experience indicates that no funding reforms should be introduced that would directly damage solidarity.

Where countries in transition to a market economy are switching to social insurance-based financing, the introduction of such a system should be done with care, to ensure that the complex institutional and technological structures required to manage a new system really do function as they should.

> **MARKETS AND HEALTH CARE**
>
> Available evidence from both western and eastern Europe indicates that unfettered markets are not compatible with the nature of health as a social good. Market mechanisms in health care are likely to be more successful, financially and operationally, if they are focused on hospitals and physicians; in contrast, efforts to create competition among multiple private insurers or to require increased co-payments from patients have been notably less successful.
>
> For the application of market mechanisms to service providers to work well, the State needs to steer and regulate these relationships. While the mix of public/private ownership of provider institutions varies greatly across Europe, both efficiency and equity require consistent and stable State regulation.
>
> *Source*: Saltman, R.B & Figueras, J. *European health care reform. Analysis of current strategies*. Copenhagen, WHO Regional Office for Europe, 1997 (WHO Regional Publications, European Series, No. 72).

Resource allocation according to need

The evidence suggests that a strategic approach to resource allocation and priority-setting is needed, in order to coordinate decision-making at different levels, and this should start with a discussion and a decision on the values and principles to be applied when determining need and selecting priorities. A debate (involving government, health service and care providers, the public and patients) on the ethical, political and social questions that need to be addressed must precede any decision on the rationing of resources. Any rationing of access to necessary services should be preceded by a thorough scrutiny of the overall organization and of the cost and effectiveness of the services and care provided.

Needs-based resource allocation formulae have been introduced into some countries in the western part of the Region and are now being developed in some countries in the eastern part, in particular regarding the geographical allocation of resources and services.

Contracting is a mechanism that offers an alternative to traditional models of resource allocation, binding third-party payers and providers to explicit commitments and generating the economic motivation to meet these commitments. Four major reasons have been put forward for introducing contractual relationships into tax-based systems, based on the long experience of health insurance systems:

- to encourage decentralization
- to improve the performance of providers
- to improve the planning of health service and care development
- to improve management.

Contracts can support equity if, through needs assessment, resources are allocated as a priority explicitly to disadvantaged population groups. The role of governments should be to ensure equity, in order to avoid over-emphasizing profitable, rather than effective, services.

Provider payments to create incentives for quality

Paying primary health care providers

Payment systems for PHC providers should contribute to achievement of the best possible health outcomes. An optimum payment system for PHC providers should also ensure the following: financial management of the different components of PHC within a country's total health care expenditure; a balanced package of health promotion, disease prevention, treatment, and rehabilitative services; a free choice of health care provider (nurse, physician, hospital) for all individuals; a structure of fair rewards for practitioners which recognizes workload and professional merit; acceptance of health care providers' responsibility for and accountability to the population and responsiveness to the needs of the community, the family and the individual; promotion of close collaboration among health care providers; and a democratic system of decision-making. Finally, the system should allow purposeful, flexible management aimed at achieving continuous quality development and greater cost–effectiveness.

Mixed payment systems, with a prospective component based on capitation together with fee-for-service for selected items, seem to be more successful in controlling costs at the macro level, while ensuring both patient and provider satisfaction and achieving efficiency and quality at the micro level. The tools available for management include the use of different incentives to influence patterns of care (e.g. to offer more preventive services) and ensure equitable distribution of primary care providers throughout the country.

Paying for secondary and tertiary care

Prospective budgeting has evident merits: it limits expenditure to funding a given level of service provision that is determined in advance for a defined period. A prospective budgeting system can be recommended if it incorporates the use of case-mix controls and output measures. Classification systems based on diagnosis or on the characteristics of the patients can be used to better analyse cost structures, evaluate hospital performance and quality of care, and make comparisons between hospitals in terms of costs and quality, as well as in negotiating contracts between hospitals and those purchasing services.

Alternatively, a volume-based approach can be made to work by using prospective pricing and contracting or planning agreements for agreed levels of service provision. In this way, hospitals can be obliged to achieve specific objectives of cost control and effective resource utilization, stimulating them to review and adjust their current organization, staffing levels and internal resource allocation.

6.4.2 Human resources

With some 1.5 million physicians, over 4.5 million nurses and tens of millions of other health care workers in the Region, human resources are a critical factor in all health services, as they are central for policy and programme implementation. Various trends have been observed throughout the Region. The eastern and southern parts of the Region have long had health services that are overstaffed, yet unemployment and other market forces have done little to reduce the supply of physicians. In spite of overstaffing, a number of countries are still experiencing difficulties in staffing rural areas. In many Member States, the shortage of appropriately skilled family health doctors and nurses and other PHC staff is a serious problem, while the education of health professionals has become out of balance, too often producing over-specialized physicians and under-qualified nurses. It is oriented towards disease alone, rather than to disease and health, and it is confined to the hospital setting or even limited to highly specialized tertiary care. Health promotion and disease prevention are usually undervalued. Furthermore, the education which different health professionals undergo is often completely separate, and they do not come together during their training, so, teamwork is generally not promoted.

Education has traditionally paid too little attention to those elements of professionals' work that are vital for population-based health. These "missing" elements include epidemiologically based needs assessment, the principles and practice of health promotion, disease prevention and rehabilitative care, and the systematic measurement and analysis of the quality of their own work. Continuing professional education is in general poorly developed.

TARGET 18 – DEVELOPING HUMAN RESOURCES FOR HEALTH

BY THE YEAR 2010, ALL MEMBER STATES SHOULD HAVE ENSURED THAT HEALTH PROFESSIONALS AND PROFESSIONALS IN OTHER SECTORS HAVE ACQUIRED APPROPRIATE KNOWLEDGE, ATTITUDES AND SKILLS TO PROTECT AND PROMOTE HEALTH.

In particular:

18.1 the education of health professionals should be based on the principles of the HFA policy, preparing them to provide promotive, preventive, curative and rehabilitative services of good quality and helping to bridge clinical and public health practice;

18.2 planning systems should be in place to ensure that the number and mix of health professionals trained meet current and future health needs;

18.3 all Member States should have adequate capacity for specialized training in public health leadership, management and practice;

18.4 the education of professionals in other sectors should include the basic principles of the HFA policy and, specifically, knowledge of how their work can influence the determinants of health.

PROPOSED STRATEGIES

Professional characteristics

Human resources for health should be adequate in number, and they should be equipped with the skills and competencies to respond to the requirements and foreseeable needs of health services. This will entail rethinking programmes for the undergraduate, postgraduate and continuing education of physicians, nurses, managers and other health care professionals. Such a review should result in the necessary changes being made to the place and content of education, so that heath professionals are fitted for carrying out the functions of modern HFA-based public health and health service practice, in which greater emphasis is placed in particular on health promotion, PHC and the quality of care.

Close collaboration with professional peers is an important element of professional work and needs to be absorbed more fully into professional ethics. In Europe this has been a tradition in hospital medicine but less frequently seen in PHC – however, working alone with no regular exchanges of experience for mutual improvement can no longer be considered professionally satisfactory. In a similar way, all those engaged in PHC, (such as nurses, pharmacists, dentists and social workers) must work in a team and recognize the need to cooperate on tackling the many complex health problems that cannot be adequately dealt with by one profession alone.

Physicians and nurses need to take responsibility for the consequences of their own lifestyles on their patients' health and to be educated accordingly. For instance, much research has demonstrated that whether or not physicians are smokers has a major impact on how active and effective they are in advising patients to stop smoking. Similarly, lifestyle counselling needs to be part of everyday practice for health care providers.

One area where health professionals need to develop their commitment and skills is the development of better quality of care. Individual health care providers need to monitor their own performance and compare it with that of their peers, as an essential ethical component of professional practice. In order to bring about such a change, professional education needs to be modified and professional organizations must strongly support it. The three European forums for medical, pharmaceutical, and nursing associations, working with WHO, have an important role to play in capturing the commitment of professional associations to these developments on a regional basis.

Integrated health care is provided by a multidisciplinary team of health professionals. During their education, all health professionals should be inspired by respect for human dignity, professional ethics and solidarity. It is important to recognize that each profession has its special area of competence and that they need to work together on the basis of mutual respect for each other's expertise. Working together does not necessarily mean working under the same roof (although that is advantageous), but knowing each other, performing complementary work, constantly exchanging information and meeting at regular intervals to facilitate cooperation. The appropriate mix of skills required for different settings should be defined and the number of training positions planned accordingly.

Planning human resources

In order to ensure that the supply of health personnel meets their needs, countries must have the capacity to plan future human resource requirements. This will require appropriately trained personnel and the necessary tools. They should also have the ongoing capacity to review and update existing plans, conduct policy analyses and prepare projections and scenarios. To this end, they need a well developed human resources management information system and a process that includes the many players involved in human resources development.

Some countries in the eastern part of the Region are characterized by too many health personnel. However, although the total number is high, some of these countries still suffer from uneven distribution of staff. A rationalization in the total number is generally planned as a means of improving efficiency and matching the most appropriate service providers to the service needs of the population. This rationalization can be ensured by a combination of several measures – reductions in force through restrictions in the supply of trained staff, revised staffing norms, redistribution of existing staff and rational deployment in the future through better management.

Training of health professionals

The education of health professionals should be designed in accordance with the health needs of society and aimed at ensuring that they acquire the necessary knowledge and skills. All settings where health care is provided, such as homes, schools, workplaces, primary care settings and hospitals, should be integrated into education as key learning environments. The education of health professionals at different levels – undergraduate, postgraduate and continuing education – should be strongly interlinked to create a continuous process. The strategies and content of education at the different levels should be defined accordingly.

Health professionals should be educated to possess well developed analytical, communication and managerial skills. In particular, they have to be strong problem-solvers and able both to work in teams and to understand social and cultural realities. Education systems should foster the active participation of students in the learning process. Assessment of the quality of education should be based on the students' knowledge, skills, attitudes and abilities. Evaluation of graduates' performance a certain time after they have started their practical work could yield valuable feedback information for further improving educational objectives and curricula.

The teaching staff are active facilitators of learning, rather than merely transferring knowledge. To perform this role, teaching staff need opportunities to update their knowledge, and they need to have the flexibility to adapt themselves to new teaching techniques.

Physicians need to be able to diagnose the health problems of individuals and society, to protect individuals and society from disease, to promote health and, when necessary, to treat and rehabilitate individuals and society. They should therefore be educated in management principles relating to cost–effectiveness, efficient use of resources and appropriate technologies, and in essential aspects of the economic and social sciences relevant to health.

Human resources for primary health care

The multidisciplinary team of health professionals working in PHC settings includes physicians, nurses, midwives, feldshers, dentists, pharmacists, physiotherapists, social workers, etc. However, special reference will be made here to the qualifications of the physicians and nurses working in PHC settings, since they are the two professions which are at the hub of the network of services.

The primary care physician must be trained in providing services to the entire population irrespective of age, gender, social class, race or religion and covering the whole range of conditions that present themselves in PHC, without excluding any category of complaint or health problem that might be encountered. GPs should therefore, have a family health profile, being able to recognize problems in terms of their patients' physical, psychological and social perspectives, and in particular those that are related to their family circumstances or to deficiencies in their social support. The education of physicians should ensure that they acquire the necessary knowledge and skills to do this. Whether the general practitioner/family health physician will be a specialist or possess the skills to carry out these functions straight after graduating from medical school is a question currently being debated in a number of countries. While that decision will have to be made in accordance with the specific conditions of each country, two points are crucial: on the one hand, the physician should fulfil the minimum requirements in terms of knowledge and abilities, and on the other hand, status (which, in professional medical circles, usually accompanies the award of a specialist degree) is important to ensure that both the population and the hospital sector regard the primary care level as the competent and important service it must be allowed to be.

A well trained family health nurse, as recommended by the 1988 Vienna Conference on Nursing, is another key PHC professional who can make a very substantial contribution to health promotion and disease prevention, besides being a care giver. Family health nurses can help individuals and families to cope with illness and chronic disability, or during times of stress, by spending a large part of their time working in patients' homes and with their families. Such nurses give advice on lifestyle and behavioural risk factors, as well as assisting families with matters concerning health. Through prompt detection, they can ensure that the health problems of families are treated at an early stage. With their knowledge of public health and social issues and other social agencies, they can identify the effects of socioeconomic factors on a family's health and refer them to the appropriate agency. They can facilitate the early discharge of people from hospital by providing nursing care at home, and they can act as the lynchpin between the family and the family health physician, substituting for the physician when the identified needs are more relevant to nursing expertise.

Health service managers

The trends towards decentralization and management flexibility, greater autonomy for all health care establishments and the introduction of regulated markets have all made managerial skills a key issue, since these processes require greater sophistication in management skills than was the case with the hierarchical administrative systems of the past.

In addition, the concept of regionalization (whereby individual health care facilities are assigned responsibility for identifying and responding to the health needs of a specific population) requires managers of such facilities to have received some education in public health, including epidemiology, so that they are familiar with needs assessment, health programming and outcome monitoring techniques. Programmes are required which will prepare personnel with an appropriate mix of skills both to carry out strategic planning and to run institutions, while all categories of health professionals need to be better able to lead, negotiate and communicate in a sector where dealing with other people is a constant feature. (The management of the sector is dealt with in more detail in section 6.5 below.)

Management of human resources

Management of human resource for health implies that personnel are utilized in a manner that is consistent with their competencies under conditions that promote effective work. It also covers the geographical distribution of health staff in the country and the relationship to the population and their health service needs.

In order to ensure that a country's investment in human resources is protected, it is necessary for the recruitment process to be carried out as thoroughly and as methodically as possible. Sound recruitment and retention policies are a prerequisite for an effective workforce.

Sometimes professional qualifications are set too high and too rigidly imposed for the tasks to be done – there is scope for staff to perform more tasks and to substitute for other professionals. The minimum requirements for any promotion (qualifications, experience, etc.) also need to be set according to the capabilities required.

There are a number of other factors that will affect the behaviour of human resources. The concept of performance-related pay is a useful tool when used together with the relevant systems, measures and indicators. The financial budgeting system also needs to be designed to allow managers to offer incentives to health personnel. The impact of incentives on the behaviour of providers needs to be continuously assessed.

A good staff performance appraisal system is critical to good management of human resources. It is a prerequisite for the introduction of performance-related pay. It is also closely linked to the processes of staff development.

The issue of career development is an important one, because it affects the performance of staff and therefore the delivery of services. Career paths needs to be transparent and allow for lateral as well as upward moves. The system should apply to all levels of health personnel. In many cases, primary care teams, by the nature of their work, do not have a dynamic career path. Therefore this group of providers must be given the opportunity to take on other responsibilities, such as participation in research and teaching.

6.4.3 Pharmaceuticals

Medicines, when used appropriately, are one of the most cost-effective health care interventions. In European countries, between 10% and 30% of health care expenditure goes on medicines, but at the same time in many countries scarce resources are wasted on drugs of little or questionable usefulness and on unnecessary drug use. Pharmaceutical policies in all countries are shaped not only by public health interests but also by economic considerations, the agendas of professional bodies, consumer's behaviour and the pharmaceutical industry. In all European countries, the state has the responsibility for regulating the entry of drug products onto the market, but compliance with and enforcement of the corresponding legislation is often unsatisfactory; in some countries, drugs are imported and sold without the necessary professional control and guidance, and substandard drug products are currently a problem in several countries of the Region.

In NIS in particular, access to pharmaceuticals is seriously hampered by the economic hardships which the population are facing and the non-availability of drugs on the market, together with under-financed and unsustainable health insurance and reimbursement schemes.

In order to provide quality health care at an affordable cost, it is imperative that no funds are wasted on drugs of doubtful effectiveness, unnecessary prescribing or unnecessarily expensive medicines. European countries are already applying a mix of regulatory, administrative, financial, educational and information strategies. Measures include positive and negative lists of drugs for reimbursement; restrictions on prescribing and levels of dispensing; prescription auditing; promotion of generics; and financial controls such as patient co-payments, fixed or indicative budgets for prescribers, price regulation and reference pricing.

PROPOSED STRATEGIES

The state has an important responsibility for setting standards and regulating the efficacy, safety and quality of medicinal products, as well as for guaranteeing that the whole population has access to needed medicines.

Pharmaceutical policies should focus on enhancing access to essential drugs and making best use of public and private expenditure, in order to provide quality health care through good drug treatment at an affordable cost. This entails:

- selecting the drugs to be used on the criteria of efficacy, safety and quality, and using cost–effectiveness criteria for reimbursed drugs. WHO's essential drugs concept and the WHO revised drug strategy provide good starting points for doing this;
- securing sustainable sources of financing;
- organizing efficient and professionally responsible drug supply and delivery systems (whether public and/or private) which ensure that pharmaceuticals are accessible to those who need them;
- implementing strategies that support and reinforce the rational use of drugs.

New drug products should only enter the market if they meet the criteria of efficacy, safety and quality. When selecting a drug for inclusion in the reimbursement system, much greater emphasis needs to be placed on whether it truly has a measurably beneficial impact on the health outcome, whether it is superior to other treatments, and whether (from the health care perspective) it really needs to be paid for through public collective funds. The true impact of drug treatment on health outcome can only be assessed after several years, and this evaluation needs to be a continuous process. Information technology in post-market surveillance and pharmaco-epidemiology can provide the tools for better assessment and subsequent decision-making on these issues.

Policies should also be implemented to develop new drugs for unmet therapeutic needs.

Significant improvements in drug selection and use can be achieved by giving health professionals access to objective and impartial information on drugs and by bringing together clinicians, clinical pharmacologists and (clinical) pharmacists in pharmacotherapeutic committees in hospitals and ambulatory care settings. This requires active cooperation by all partners in health, including medical and pharmaceutical associations, the pharmaceutical industry, and consumers' and patients' groups. These groups play a vital role in enhancing the appropriate use of medicines and ensuring public and professional confidence in policy objectives and strategies.

Drug use can result in better health outcome only when patients are truly involved in and well informed about their condition and the goals of drug treatment. Health professionals have an increasing role to play in informing patients about the appropriate use of medicines. New information technology has great potential in this regard and needs to be further exploited.

PARTNERSHIP TO SAFEGUARD CONSUMERS' RIGHTS IN POLAND

In October 1994, the Polish Consumer Federation (PCF) launched an initiative with Health Action International to promote the rational use of drugs in Poland. In contrast with the shortages of drugs prior to 1989, it was found that there were now too many drugs, many of which were obsolete, ineffective, expensive and potentially harmful. The project's main goals were consumer education and increasing consumers' awareness of their rights. Initially, difficulties were experienced in securing the support of health professionals. Some physicians felt that decisions regarding drugs should be left exclusively to them. Pharmacists tended to be more supportive of the initiative.

A pamphlet *Consumers and drugs* was produced which contained information on the rational use of drugs and problem drugs on the market. The brochures were distributed to those responsible for developing and implementing national drug policies. The second step was to produce further information, entitled *Med sense* – which aimed to engender a more critical attitude among consumers towards drug promotion. The education strategy was heavily supported by television campaigns, print media and radio exposure. The project ended in 1995, with a seminar on rational drug use which brought together consumers and professionals to discuss the drug situation. The most visible success of the project was the high media exposure. Another effect was the strengthening of PCF's role so that consumers are now taken more seriously by both the pharmaceutical industry and the health sector. The Ministry of Health gave an undertaking to withdraw the most dangerous drugs from the market. Other indicators of success include:

- increased use of the WHO essential drugs list;
- instruction of medical students in good prescribing practice;
- the Institute of Psychiatry and Neurology produced a leaflet for doctors on psychotropic treatment guidelines, in order to prevent drug dependency;
- growing interest in patients' rights;
- increased media attention to rational drug use.

Source: London, Consumers' International (unpublished data).

6.4.4 Medical equipment

New health care technologies are continuously being brought to the market and affect the trends in service provision, from the points of view of both quality and cost. Practice, in relation to new technologies vary greatly throughout the Region – in many countries, new technologies are introduced without any assessment and without any plan; some countries allow the new equipment if its efficacy is proven and it will be used in a planned way, but many countries have no systematic way of assessing the relative value of new technologies over existing ones.

In the more eastern part of the Region, many countries suffer from a lack of even basic equipment, owing to economic constraints. On the other hand, some essential, basic equipment is often not available at the primary care level while much sophisticated equipment is provided in tertiary care.

PROPOSED STRATEGIES

It is essential to introduce appropriate technology on the basis of a sound assessment, and to subject new medical devices and equipment to careful assessment. Governments need to play a stronger role in regulating the introduction of new health technologies – as they have long done for pharmaceuticals. One step they could take would be to demand measurable evidence of better health and greater cost–effectiveness for new technologies compared with existing ones.

Practical experience in recent years has shown that, in spite of initial positive assessments, new health technologies are often found to be problematic when introduced widely in everyday practice. In future, the final impact on health of the routine use of new equipment should therefore be continuously monitored. Consequently, technology assessment should be seen as integral to, rather than separate from, quality of care development.

6.5 Public health infrastructure

It is essential to promote adequate capacities to manage the development and implementation of HFA-based policies and strategies; to provide an epidemiological analysis of health experience, determinants and needs; to promote programmes and activities focused on health gain; and to integrate the delivery of high-quality health care into the same population perspective. This will require a strong and sustainable political and managerial commitment.

The public health system and its infrastructure needs to be modernized and strengthened in all countries, although to different degrees. In many countries it remains institutionally and functionally weak, often with a traditional focus solely on the classic roles of public health such as communicable disease control and immunization, maternal and child health, environmental health, and the compilation of health statistics. While these remain important, the HFA approach to health development also requires the ability to take a comprehensive "horizontal" view of the needs for health improvement across society as a whole, to analyse broader strategies for health, to create innovating networks for action among many different actors and, in general, to be a catalyst for change.

Specific country experiences vary. In many Member States, the basic infrastructure provided by public health experts has declined over the past 10 to 15 years, sometimes as part of decentralization and privatization; in these countries, public health practitioners have less recognized authority than before, and their role is often challenged. In a few other countries, however, considerable public inquiry into the situation has led to stronger recognition of the important role that public health should be play within society and the health care system, and steps have already been taken to strengthen the capacity of the public health management system. Many countries of the Region need to strengthen their infrastructure for public health training.

PROPOSED STRATEGIES

To ensure development that are in line with an HFA perspective, two main categories of personnel must be considered: population-based public health managers, and other public health care workers.

6.5.1 Public health managers

The essential role of the public health function is to identify, analyse and report on health experience and its determinants. What is the pattern of disease and disability within a society, and why? This analysis and reporting is the essential preliminary to political, professional and public debate about the action by which health may be improved. Such action will certainly involve other sectors as partners with the health sector and health services. It will also involve policy and programme development at several levels (international, national, regional and local) and in a variety of settings (cities, schools, etc). What has often been lacking so far has been a sound structure for the functioning of this public health perspective, the public health function, and a close working relationship between this and individual clinical work.

Ultimately, the capacity to make the case for health and to engage people, communities, health-creating sectors, policy-makers, health care managers and professionals will depend on the skills, fortitude and authority of current and future public health practitioners and on the quality of their leadership. Such practitioners, in national, subnational and local positions, must be professionally trained in public health to postgraduate level, and they must be experienced in population-based public health work in a variety of political and administrative settings. Although the situation varies from country to country, the Region as a whole needs many more public health practitioners, trained to support population-based action to improve health, as well as an adequate institutional infrastructure for their work.

Public health practitioners need to use political awareness for the benefit of populations and mobilize broad-based political and cultural support for equitable, sustainable and accountable approaches to health development. They must be able to motivate and assist people, organizations, communities and countries to manage and adapt effectively to changing environments, as well as facilitate the development of local capacities. Furthermore, they must be able boldly and effectively to challenge groups whose activities are detrimental to the public's health.

Essentially what is needed are public health managers, with the skills to manage partnerships and coordinated multisectoral action within alliances. They must have a thorough understanding of the contribution different sectors and different partners can make to solving health problems, be trained in population-based analysis of health problems, be grounded in the approaches to deal with problems of lifestyles, the environment and health care, and be capable of the advocacy and networking needed to bring many partners together. They must also be skilled in creating excellent public health information for the general public, professionals and politicians. In these tasks they will have to be supported by a variety of experts in specific technical fields.

Within the health service itself they must be trained in policy and programme planning, including target-setting, outcome measurement and evaluation, and instrumental in shaping the pattern of services provided. They must be able to help plan, monitor and evaluate broad health development programmes, defined by disease category or client group, making scientifically informed judgements about the balance to be struck (in terms of health improvement, investment and service delivery) between health promotion, disease prevention, therapy and rehabilitation. All these are exceptionally demanding requirements for public health managers, and their education needs are accordingly considerable.

Countries should review their existing systems to see whether they have clear mandates and sufficient capacity to take such population-based public health action. It will be particularly vital to strengthen the infrastructure, capacity and profile of educational institutions – such as schools of public health – that train public health managers, and to design better common curricula. The need for change in education is particularly acute in the more easterly part of the Region, but this issue needs to be given much higher priority in the health development programmes of many countries.

6.5.2 Other public health workers

In addition to population-based public health managers, human resources for HFA and public health exist throughout society, both within and outside the health sector. These resources can be regarded as contributing in important ways to the public health function – they are thus part of the "public health infrastructure" in a broad sense of that term. Several categories may be defined:

- In broad terms, a vast potential for public health can be mobilized from many people and professionals in their daily work. They include not only doctors, nurses, pharmacists, social workers, etc., but also professionals working in schools, the media, town planning, architecture, and welfare services, as well as people involved in NGOs of many kinds.

- Many of the scientific and technical skills needed for public health practice are provided by epidemiologists, information scientists, social scientists, health economists, operational researchers, lawyers, political and administrative scientists, experts on infectious disease control, environment and health specialists, etc.

- As indicated above, health service managers need to have a more detailed understanding of population perspectives and public health issues, so that they can understand the relationship of their service (hospital, health centre) to the surrounding population. They should think in terms of the needs of the whole population served by the institution (not only the patients) and the health gain to be achieved by its services, as well as the quality and cost–effectiveness of the services delivered.

All these "public health workers" are a vital resource for health. They should receive and value education and information about health experiences and issues, in order that they can contribute to the perception of health as a positive public message throughout society, and they should play an important role in developing and carrying out multisectoral policies and programmes for health improvement.

Special HFA-based educational objectives and programme components relating to health and health improvement therefore need to be developed and tailored for use in many postgraduate and continuing education programmes. This applies to the education of economists, architects, journalists, lawyers, social workers, engineers and others outside the health sector, for example, and of all those within the sector who are identified as having a contribution to make to public health improvement.

Finally, there is a need to promote excellence in public health development by sharing knowledge. To a large extent this can be done by networking, as the networks of Regions for Health, Healthy Cities, Health Promoting Schools, Health Promoting Hospitals, Health in Prisons, CINDI, etc. have amply shown. In future it is hoped that much greater use will be made of such networks; they should be promoted as major vehicles for stimulating public health action on a countrywide basis in every Member State.

Chapter 7

Policies and mechanisms for managing change

> Target 19 – Research and knowledge for health
> Target 20 – Mobilizing partners for health
> Target 21 – Policies and strategies for health for all

7.1 Introduction

As emphasized in previous chapters, the changes that need to be made, on the basis of HFA principles, in order to improve the health of European populations extend beyond the health services to encompass the whole of society. They are conceptually and practically complex, and within the European Region the many actors involved – institutions, organizations and individuals – will need to be mobilized. This chapter considers the processes by which these resources may be brought together for health in a coordinated way, structured around HFA principles.

The bureaucratic, hierarchical organization and management systems and styles of old will not suffice to achieve these goals, and new systems for multisectoral and organizational cooperation and coordination will be required. The general public and a broad range of organizations, institutions and sectors must be informed and motivated about what needs to be done to achieve health improvement, and they must be drawn into active coalitions for health. The relevant management skills to promote change throughout complex modern, plural societies will be at a premium and will require substantial development.

This chapter considers some of the necessary dimensions of change, i.e. improving the knowledge base for planning and action through research and improved information systems (section 7.2); how to mobilize a wide range of partners to create countrywide movements for health (section 7.3); and finally, how to organize the process of HFA policy planning, implementation and evaluation (section 7.4).

7.2 Strengthening the knowledge base for health

Research – to develop better tools to protect health and treat illness – and health information systems are two key areas for change.

7.2.1 Research

All policies and actions to improve health need a firm knowledge base, and research is one of society's most valuable and important tools for laying the foundation of better strategies to improve health and health care. None the less, only a few Member States have followed the extensive advice given by the WHO European Advisory Committee on Health Research regarding the need to formulate national HFA-oriented research policies and programmes.

Basic research, in such areas as improving fundamental knowledge of biological processes, mapping the human genome and looking for new drugs to improve the treatment of disease, is currently being undertaken on a large scale in many countries of the Region, financed both from public funds and by private industry. By and large the current system functions reasonably well, although more research could be directed towards highly promising or high-priority fields, such as immunology, genetics, or refining the immunization tools by developing multi-potent vaccines that are easier, cheaper and simpler to store and distribute.

More problematic is the lack of a systematic approach to clinical research in many areas of medicine, as well as the low priority given to operational research in the health care field. Accordingly, a substantial part of both areas of current practice is not sufficiently evidence-based.

The growing role of research means the scientific community should be more involved in developing scientifically sound, socially relevant and feasible bases for decisions. In most countries, however, there must be a much better match between the needs for health research as perceived by decision-makers and planners on the one hand, and the research priorities set by the research community on the other. In addition, hardly any country today has a systematic mechanism for ensuring that new evidence from research is actually introduced into daily practice. The dialogue between the two communities therefore needs to be significantly strengthened, not just in order to make research more focused; but also, and no less important, to ensure that those responsible for services are more motivated to implement change, because they have themselves been involved in designing the research.

The European context for research initiatives related to health is now very promising. In addition to the considerable research efforts of individual Member States, it includes the EU's proposed Fifth Framework Programme and the research commissioning work of the EU's Directorate-General XII, the European Medical Research Council, the European Science Foundation, and a variety of foundations, private industry and charitable institutions, as well as WHO.

7.2.2 Health information support

Information systems are another key component making knowledge more widely available, and today the world is living in a communications era.

In the health field, many new systems have been developed to improve clinical patient care (see also section 6.3). "Telemedicine" links expert centres to other parts of the health care system in a number of countries, making it possible to transfer diagnostic information from the PHC provider or local hospital to specialized centres in tertiary hospitals, with rapid feedback of advice. Automated medical records have been developed in hospital and PHC systems. Direct electronic communication links, for example between PHC physicians and pharmacists, have simplified and accelerated some aspects of health care. Sophisticated patient monitoring systems have greatly improved emergency and intensive care. However, information feedback systems, to improve the quality of care, are as yet only in the early stages of development.

Progress in taking advantage of these developments has been very uneven. For many countries of the European Region, particularly those in the east, such new systems are only now starting to arrive and they will probably not be in widespread routine use for a considerable time yet.

For consumers, only a very limited number of health information databases are currently available, and those only in a few countries. There are no clear thoughts at the moment as to how the quality of data input can be monitored or guaranteed, to ensure that consumers get correct information that will really help them to improve their understanding of the health care system and its outcomes.

On the public health level, information on health status, risk factors and health service organization is crucial. A very important factor in this respect has been the agreement that all Member States use and report on a common set of global and European HFA indicators. This has now been operating successfully since 1984, and a large database has been developed, enabling Member States to compare data on a wide variety of health outcome and risk factors that are useful to planners and decision-makers (although data collection in individual countries can still be improved).

A number of WHO data systems dedicated to such topics as food safety and infectious disease control are now in operation. Coordination and cooperation is an issue, as the EU is also starting to develop new systems on infectious disease control and other topics for its countries. Similarly, there is a need for coordination with OECD which collects data on health care expenditure and certain other health-related elements.

Telematics services, providing information through modern communications technologies (especially computers, multimedia and telecommunications), can increasingly be used to support education for health, health care (telemedicine, early warning systems, etc.), health research and health services management.

> **TARGET 19 – RESEARCH AND KNOWLEDGE FOR HEALTH**
>
> BY THE YEAR 2005, ALL MEMBER STATES SHOULD HAVE HEALTH RESEARCH, INFORMATION AND COMMUNICATION SYSTEMS THAT BETTER SUPPORT THE ACQUISITION, EFFECTIVE UTILIZATION, AND DISSEMINATION OF KNOWLEDGE TO SUPPORT HEALTH FOR ALL.
>
> In particular:
>
> 19.1 all countries should have research policies oriented towards the priorities of their long-term policies for health for all;
>
> 19.2 all countries should have mechanisms that enable health services delivery and development to be based on scientific evidence;
>
> 19.3 health information should be useful to and easily accessible by politicians, managers, health and other professionals, as well as the general public;
>
> 19.4 all countries should have established health communication policies and programmes which support the agenda of health for all and facilitate access to such information.

PROPOSED STRATEGIES

Developing the research agenda for HFA

Most Member States need to develop a health-oriented research policy – the guidance given by the WHO European Advisory Committee on Health Research provides a good framework for that – and they should encourage the research community to respond to challenges of HFA in the twenty-first century. The systematic search for better tools of health promotion, disease prevention, diagnosis, treatment, rehabilitation and care – for use both in clinical care and in public health – should be intensified and, for each major area of health problems (such as cardiovascular disease) scientific committees should systematically analyse the scientific evidence base and feed their findings into continuously updated databases. Countries should have a mechanism for identifying the gaps in such evidence, and they should seek ways of filling those gaps with new research in areas where the knowledge base is insufficient. There is also a need to develop new approaches to deal with broader societal changes, such as socioeconomic deprivation, differences in health between the sexes, etc.

Special efforts should be made to develop research for anticipating future trends, needs and challenges in health, covering not only direct indicators of health but also indicators of structural, environmental, behavioural and social determinants.

As health services account for 5–10% of GNP and employ 5–8% of the total workforce in countries, it is increasingly important to carry out research on health care reform alternatives and their true impact. Thus, no new health care reform should be launched unless it includes a clear evaluation component, so that it will be possible to "learn from doing".

The public sector and the scientific community should cooperate on setting research priorities, and the mechanisms for dialogue and cooperation between policy- and decision-makers and the scientific community need to be significantly strengthened through special committees, earmarked research funds, joint participation in research, etc.

One very important task for virtually every Member State in the Region is to establish a permanent mechanism that will make a systematic review – e.g. once a year – of all major national and international research outcomes in the main areas of health development (TB, cancer, drug use, etc.). Such a review should identify all the major findings that ought to be introduced into daily practice in the country concerned and bring them to the attention of the highest decision-making level in the health sector. As mentioned in Chapter 2, this would also be helpful to the idea of establishing a "WHO country function" in every Member State.

International research collaboration at the European level should be strengthened, with greater emphasis placed on needs-based research, an increase in the number of intercountry research programmes and better exchange of research information. For example, the European Commission, the European Science Foundation and WHO should work more closely together on research; a good start has been made on the environment and health, but closer cooperation is also required in many other health fields.

Developing health information support

Health information must become much more widely available and easily accessible, if HFA is to be properly understood and actively promoted. Decision-makers, health professionals, economists, architects, teachers, research workers, the media, the general public, etc. all need to be informed about health issues in a way which arouses both their interest in and commitment to the implications and processes of health improvement.

One way of doing this is to strengthen the mechanisms for monitoring health and its known determinants, as well as the operation of the health care system. For this purpose, countries should use the global and regional HFA indicators, as a minimum – and preferably augmented by specific ones reflecting each country's own HFA targets. This information should be available on electronic media and be published regularly in a publicly accessible form, so as to promote an informed and open debate among politicians, professionals and the public concerning health outcomes and determinants, and future priorities for action and investment.

Data should be specifically adapted to, and presented at, each of the major levels (country, subnational, local community, institution) that are chosen for the planning and implementation of HFA programmes (see section 7.4 below).

The European HFA indicators will be updated to reflect the changing priorities that will emerge from the current update of the regional HFA policy and targets (see Annex 2). Some aspects relating to health outcomes need further strengthening, in particular with regard to risk factors.

Here a European standard for periodic health surveys is needed, to improve the information provided to individual countries and the Region as a whole on lifestyle and health risk factors. A WHO model – European health interview survey (EUROHIS) – is currently being developed. Similarly, further strengthening of communicable disease, food safety and environment and health surveillance networks and indicators is desirable. Such strengthening will involve greater standardization of definitions and data collection systems in all Member States.

Ensuring free access by users, including the general public, to databases that draw attention to European health problems, risk factors, measures to deal with them, and the grounds for health care action will be an important task in the coming decades. One particularly important issue is the development of special databases for the general public providing useful information on self-care.

WHO has started work on quality indicators and databases for use at clinical level by physicians, nurses and other health care providers, but this needs to be further pursued. This work should include preparation of internationally agreed quality indicators – a WHO responsibility – and a system of interlinked databases that provide feedback of results to individual users so that they can compare themselves with their peers. It will be important to ensure confidentiality of both patients and care providers in clinical-level databases, in order to enhance the validity of the information entered. Aggregated, anonymized information should, however, be made available for management purposes at institutional and population-based levels. A number of pilot areas in the European Region are now incorporated in a WHO system of linked databases that permit the use of standardized quality indicators to compare outcomes of care.

Measures to ensure that local populations are better informed about health, lifestyle and environment problems and development activities in their local communities are a prerequisite for community involvement and participation, and they should be developed with imagination and innovation. Current examples include the use of conventional media, as well as new opportunities created by electronic communication. Again the media and communication sector has a vital role to play in informing, educating and persuading people about their individual and collective responsibility for health, as well as about the options for action.

Telematics

The wider use of telematics in public health and patient care will be a very important strategy for Member States, and one that can help bring expert knowledge to new areas and institutions in a cost-effective and rapid manner. However, such a strategy should take into account a number of elements:[18]

---

[18] Adapted from: *A health telematics policy in support of WHO's Health-for-All strategy for global health development: report of the WHO Consultation on Health Telematics, Geneva, 11–17 December 1997.* Geneva, World Health Organization, 1998.

- health telematics systems and services should be dictated by health needs and by clinical and public health standards, not be technology-driven;
- the values and principles of HFA, notably equity, sustainability, participation and accountability, should apply fully to the development of health telematics;
- health telematics requires new skills from the relevant decision-makers, operators and users, calling for a mix of participatory education, skills training, continuing professional education and lifelong learning;
- given the fast rate of technological obsolescence and changing price–performance ratios, countries will benefit from closer collaboration on the development of technological standards, compatibility, open architecture, competitive prices and pilot applications.

Managing health information developments in an effective and rational way at the level of the European Region will require the major organizations active in this field to enter into more formal agreements of cooperation than is the case today; most importantly, this will involve WHO, the European Commission and OECD.

7.3 Mobilizing partners for health

As shown in Chapter 5, a wide range of partners in society need to be involved if multisectoral societal policies and actions are to be developed and harnessed for health. More specifically, section 5.4 emphasized the need to do this in order to promote healthy lifestyles, while Chapter 6 underlined the involvement not only of health professionals but also of many other partners in health care. Thus HFA means mobilizing a wide range of partners in a number of settings of daily life and at different levels of management – from the country as a whole to the local community.

The new focus on tackling the determinants of health shows that there are a number of new players who are not fully recognized as partners for health today. Many of these potential partners are not aware of the benefits they can gain from working with the health sector and investing in the health of their clients. There is therefore a need to overcome the problems posed by single-sector approaches and specific organizational objectives, budgets and activities; one of these problems is the lack of mechanisms to bring partners together in systematic cooperation.

In Chapter 1, the right to participation was advanced as one of the three fundamental HFA values. It applies to all partners for health, i.e. all those in society who, through their personal contribution as individuals or in their professional roles, can contribute to health improvement. However, with the right to participate comes the duty to be accountable (see also Chapter 1); partnership therefore, implies that all partners must take responsibility for the health consequences of their policies and actions and assume their share of accountability for health.

Governments remain fundamental partners. A central purpose of the processes of government is to enhance the human development of the population served. This is implicit in the structures of government, which have functions relating to health, education, social welfare and environmental protection, alongside economic development. However, this principle is too seldom explicit enough, and it certainly does not currently appear at the heart of economic policy-making and activity.

In the European Region, the nature and role of governments is slowly changing, moving away from the direct provision of services and support for populations towards the establishment of a framework of societal objectives and regulation within which there exist many providers, both public and private. There has also been a move to decentralize, with responsibilities being increasingly left to regional or local structures. Governments, however, still bear the ultimate responsibility for the health of their people, and for the use and outcomes of overall resources for health and health care.

Both national parliamentarians and local politicians in Europe need to put health higher on their political agendas and to be accountable for the health results achieved and the effectiveness of the health action taken. They have an indispensable role to play in providing the medium- and longer-term vision that can create more fundamental, effective and sustained results for health; when they do so, they will also realize the great potential for political support that such initiatives will create.

The various actors in the public health infrastructure – from staff at the ministry of health down to the local community public health director – have a key role to play as catalysts for action, technical experts, advisers to politicians, "networkers", etc. In the past, however, in many countries they have not – with notable exceptions – been active enough in reaching out to other sectors, nor in helping clinical medicine apply an epidemiological approach to the quality of care dilemma. More recently, innovative projects such as Healthy Cities have shown a new way forward, at the same times as expanding the notion of the public health infrastructure (see section 6.5).

Health professionals are key participants in a broad range of health actions, both as providers of services and as planners and managers of many parts of the health sector. However, their great potential has not been fully utilized in the past, since both individual health professionals and their organizations have often – again, with notable exceptions – been too narrowly focused, not looking far enough beyond individual patient care to analyse population impact. They have also often lacked the will to recognize the importance of their own function as a role model for local societies, e.g. regarding personal smoking habits. There has often been considerable reluctance to accept a health promotion role (as opposed to that of patient care) and to working with structures and sectors outside their own institutions.

However, the last decade has seen the emergence of a more public health-oriented view. The Europe-wide forums of WHO and national medical associations, national nurses' associations and national associations of pharmacy owners/pharmacists have played an important pioneering role in their development.

Educators – from kindergarten through school to university – have great potential for contributing to people's development and maintenance of HFA values, knowledge and skills. Today, however, such input rarely forms part of a carefully designed, integrated and mutually supportive programme that is systematically planned to be sustainable over the whole life course of an individual.

Researchers have key roles to play in improving the thousands of tools that the HFA needs. However, as mentioned above (section 7.2), their input is often not sufficiently focused on – or interactive with – the real priority concerns of the health care system.

The number of NGOs working in the health field is growing rapidly in Europe, particularly in western Europe. In the more eastern part of the Region (CCEE and NIS) there are as yet relatively few NGOs, although their numbers are increasing. There is a great need to stimulate and support NGO development, but without threatening their autonomy or their essential flexibility and capacity for innovation. NGOs, since they are usually less affected by organizational and bureaucratic constraints than more formally constituted international organizations, can often respond to situations faster and more flexibly.

The private sector (see section 5.5) is a vital partner for health. So far, there has often been too little appreciation of its great potential – in industry, trade, the media and elsewhere – to contribute to the strategies and processes of health improvement. Certainly the private sector is now increasingly recognizing consumers' growing demands for and concerns about health, quality of life and the broader social good, and it is making more stringent assessments of the health impact of new products.

Individuals are partners for health in two ways. First they are partners, in a private capacity, in actions which directly affect their own health and/or that of their family and friends. Second, they may be partners through membership of NGOs or participation in local community health programmes.

TARGET 20 – MOBILIZING PARTNERS FOR HEALTH

BY THE YEAR 2005, IMPLEMENTATION OF POLICIES FOR HEALTH FOR ALL SHOULD ENGAGE INDIVIDUALS, GROUPS AND ORGANIZATIONS THROUGHOUT THE PUBLIC AND PRIVATE SECTORS, AND CIVIL SOCIETY, IN ALLIANCES AND PARTNERSHIPS FOR HEALTH.

In particular:
- 20.1 the health sector should engage in active promotion and advocacy for health, encouraging other sectors to join in multisectoral activities and share goals and resources;
- 20.2 structures and processes should exist at international, country, regional and local levels to facilitate harmonized collaboration of all actors and sectors in health development.

PROPOSED STRATEGIES

Partnerships for health will be required at different levels: international, country, regional and local. They are needed for the formulation of health policy; for increasing people's perception and understanding of health issues; for developing the political will for action; for target-setting; for carrying out policies and programmes and shaping service delivery, including the selection of priorities and resource allocation; and for monitoring and evaluation of outcomes.

7.3.1 Governments

It is ultimately a government's responsibility to define and be accountable for a clear health policy for the whole country. In a European Region poised to enter the twenty-first century, governments should reflect a shift in societal values such that economic growth becomes only one objective among many – to be balanced with others, such as health advancement, sustainability, equity, social cohesion and environmental quality. In undertaking this task, governments will increasingly have to recognize the need for full participation by a wider range of partners, and for transparency in the processes of policy development.

Governments need to establish effective and permanent coordination machinery, such as a national health council, comprising senior representatives of many ministries and other partners, to ensure that a coherent approach is taken to health improvement policies and that health objectives are properly balanced in both political and technical forms. However, ministries of health must provide the main technical dimensions of health policies and shoulder the main responsibility for their implementation. To help them do this, they ought to follow and analyse more systematically national and international developments (see section 7.2), leading to better strategies and methods for action for health. The establishment of a "WHO country function" (see section 2.1) with formal links to national research bodies could contribute to, and profit from, such an initiative.

7.3.2 Politicians

Politicians, at community, regional or country levels, need a thorough analysis of the health challenges and opportunities for the populations they serve, and the European HFA policy offers them a broad strategic canvas from which to paint a similar policy at the level for which they are responsible. Their accountability for that policy should be ensured – for instance, by setting broad targets for attainment and ensuring monitoring and evaluation of the follow-through. They should also ensure that the laws and regulations they make and the economic and other incentives they offer to different sectors and institutions are truly supportive of health and, where necessary, are backed up by health impact assessment schemes.

7.3.3 Professionals

Health professionals

As the key providers of health care, health professionals and their organizations should adopt the principles of quality of care and actively facilitate the self-care of their patients (as outlined in section 6.3). Furthermore, they should accept the responsibility for adopting a healthy lifestyle that their role model status imposes on them (see section 6.4.2). Finally, their technical expertise gives them particular responsibility for supporting local community and national health development programmes.

Public health professionals

Their role and responsibilities have been dealt with extensively in section 6.5.

Other professionals

Many professionals outside the health sector can be regarded as "other public health workers" within the wider public health infrastructure (see section 6.5).

Teachers in both kindergartens and schools have three important challenges to meet:

- First, they need to acquire the knowledge and teaching skills to educate and inspire their pupils to respect the basic values of fairness, equity, compassion and sustainable development. It is vital to encourage pupils to adopt healthy lifestyles and train them to resist peer pressure; teach them life skills so that they can cope with stress and adversity in a mature way; prepare them for the challenges of adolescence; instil in them the value of social interaction and the importance of social networks; and help prepare them eventually to become good parents themselves.
- Second, teachers must recognize and accept responsibility for the fact that they are important role models for their pupils, adopting healthy lifestyles (e.g. nonsmoking), and displaying the ability to cope well with stress.
- Third, teachers should recognize the need to understand better the family situation of their pupils and reach out to parents in a spirit of partnership (see section 5.4).

Engineers, architects and town planners need to broaden their understanding of the impact which their work can have on the health of individuals and communities. They should not only be aware of safety concerns relevant to the design of housing, neighbourhoods and cities, but also look for imaginative new solutions that will for example stimulate a moderate amount of daily physical exercise, promote the development of neighbourhood-based social networks, provide housing that three generations can live in, and promote the extended family as a means of breaking down the social isolation of many of today's modern urban environments.

Economists should increasingly consider not only health care resources and inputs, but also the health outcomes and services produced by the health care system and its different components. For example, it will be necessary to look more critically at the health and social costs of industrial and infrastructure development projects. One way forward would be to offer earmarked financial incentives, for example from a special Health Fund paid for by tobacco taxes, to improve functions such as health promotion and quality of care.

More vigorous and open involvement of journalists and other professionals working in the media and the communication industry in creating and sustaining public knowledge and debate about health issues will be vital to the success of HFA policy, with its emphasis on public participation and the transparency of policy-making and implementation processes. Special training in such health issues should be part of the education of such professionals. The health sector itself must make a start by welcoming a more open dialogue on its affairs.

7.3.4 Nongovernmental organizations

NGOs are essential partners for health; they are a vital component of a modern civil society, raising people's awareness of issues and their concerns, advocating change and creating a dialogue on policy; and their role in health should be strengthened. They can provide significant health and social care services to complement those of the public and private sectors, thus mobilizing important untapped resources. In particular, their role in fostering self-help, i.e. in helping people suffering from a specific health problem (such as haemophiliacs, diabetics, drug and alcohol users) to take better care of themselves, should be strongly supported. However, the strengths and potential of NGOs need to be more closely coordinated with organized public efforts at community or national level to improve the health of population groups. In this NGOs must be seen as true partners. Their involvement in local health programmes also offers an excellent example of local democracy in action– a particularly valuable characteristic for countries in transition – and great potential for releasing local resources for health by mobilizing strong local community support.

For WHO, a key current priority is to set up more flexible and inclusive mechanisms for creating and sustaining a dialogue with NGOs. This would open up the possibility of combining WHO's knowledge of the overall needs and options relating to health with the capacities of NGOs for close identification with the issues and the people involved.

7.3.5 Private sector

The private sector should listen more carefully to consumers, critically assess how its products can promote health and contribute to a better environment. There will be increasing requests for scientific evidence in support of statements of product benefit, and for the use of objective tools such as health impact assessments. Accordingly, private sector activities should become more comprehensive and health-focused than they are today. Furthermore, the private sector is a vital component of communities at both local and national levels; its support should therefore be actively sought for the development and implementation of public health programmes, as partners and in full recognition of its potentially crucial contribution.

As mentioned in section 5.4, the workplace is one of the most effective settings in which to help adults adopt healthier lifestyles. It is therefore vital that the private sector pays close attention to the health of its employees. One way forward would be to promote the concept of a "healthy company or enterprise", based on partnership between employers, employees and occupational health services. This should comprise a three-pronged approach: the creation of a healthy workforce, the production of healthy company products, and active support by the company to local community (or national) health programmes. Such action should itself be supported by national employers' and employees' associations and by the public health sector; it could build, over time, towards the establishment of a "healthy company" network.

7.3.6 Individual citizens

Making healthy choices the easier choices, through the actions outlined in previous chapters (Chapter 5 in particular), is a vital strategy for helping people to accept more responsibility for the "healthiness" of their own lives, recognizing health as a resource to be protected and actively enhanced. Similarly, individuals should accept responsibility for helping friends and relatives to choose and maintain healthy lifestyles, both by setting a personal example and through direct support.

7.3.7 Bringing partners together for action

For a strategy of partnership in health development to be truly effective, special mechanisms must be established to ensure the focus and sustainability of the partnerships. Based on the HFA policy many countries have recently made great strides in developing such partnership through movements such as Healthy Cities, Health Promoting Schools, Health Promoting Hospitals, Health in Prisons, etc. (see section 5.4). What is needed now is a strategy and structural mechanisms for mobilizing such partnerships for health throughout society.

Homes

The informal setting of the family environment does not require formal mechanisms, but a highly-respected family health nurse can be very effective in initiating constructive discussions among family members on their health challenges. A well planned family health physician concept – including family-based epidemiology and record-keeping that permits team reviews (e.g. by a physician, nurse and social worker), when needed, of families with special health or social needs – can also make a big difference.

Schools, worksites, etc.

As mentioned in section 5.4, kindergartens, schools, prisons, etc. are important settings for health action. They require a health promotion committee, provided with meaningful resources for action, composed of the major partners, and given clear responsibility to promote local health.

Local communities

The tasks of designing an HFA-oriented community health policy, complete with targets and an action programme, and of executing, monitoring and evaluating its implementation, are vital components of the HFA approach that must be tackled on a properly planned basis by every local community in every Member State (see sections 5.4 and 7.4). For this to happen, there must be a local health council or similar body charged with this responsibility and involving the elected local council, representatives of major sectors such as health, education, social affairs, etc., and the principal NGOs, the media and the local population (the latter through public hearings, for example). The local public health officer and other public health practitioners have vital technical and leadership functions to perform here.

National and subnational levels

The formulation of a countrywide HFA-oriented policy and programme remains indispensable, in order to establish a medium-term development framework with clear HFA targets that can inspire synergistic efforts and point out a common direction for similar efforts at other levels in the country (see below, section 7.4). This is also needed to ensure the rational use of resources throughout the country and to facilitate a society-wide movement towards better health that is actively supported by all ministries, national professional associations, organizations of labour and industry, the media and others.

As mentioned above, it is indispensable to have a clear, visible mechanism, such as a national health council, to develop this collective commitment. Such a council should receive technical support and leadership from the ministry of health. It should be the body to draft national policies and programmes, to monitor and evaluate the implementation of such policies and programmes, and to report on progress. This process will help create public accountability, heightening awareness of health development goals throughout society and generating the will to achieve them.

European regional level

For the 51 countries of the European Region, a permanent collaborative mechanism already exists in the WHO Regional Committee for Europe, the "parliament for health" that brings together ministers of health for an annual review of health policies and programmes in the Region. The European regional HFA policy represents their policy and targets for joint, Region-wide action, as well as an inspirational framework for individual countries to build on. The Region-wide use of the HFA targets and the HFA evaluation process (currently performed every six years) ensures public transparency and systematic feedback; the findings are all taken into account when the European HFA policy is periodically updated (every six to seven years).

Partnership with other major integrational and intergovernmental bodies is of the utmost importance if health is to be achieved across Europe. Such bodies include the European Union, the

World Bank, the Council of Europe, OECD and various humanitarian and development agencies within the United Nations system. While all are paying increasing attention to health in their policy-making and activities, the increased public health competence of the EU, and the World Bank's recent development of strategic policy in the fields of health, population and nutrition, are particularly worthy of note. There have been many significant developments in building closer collaboration between all these organizations, but much further progress can be made and more formal partnership agreements, in particular between WHO, the European Commission and the Council of Europe, would be helpful. Chapter 1 outlines the five major roles which the WHO Regional Office for Europe should play in European health development.

One example of successful partnership-building has been in the area of environmental health, where the creation of a European Environment and Health Committee has resulted in a structure that provides for frequent discussions of major policy and programme issues, leading to closer cooperation and better understanding among all the major organizations involved. As a further example, the Health Promoting Schools project brings together the European Commission, the Council of Europe and the WHO Regional Office in a practical, long-term and innovative partnership.

Attempts to bring professional and institutional partners together in a Europe-wide HFA movement have been remarkably successful. As already mentioned, a European Forum of National Medical Associations and WHO now includes representatives from national medical associations in almost all Member States, and the EuroPharm Forum for the pharmaceutical professions comprises some two thirds of all Member States. Both of these organizations will continue to take up key HFA challenges such as quality of care, and lifestyle and health issues, not only through their annual conferences but also through more permanent action-oriented task forces. In 1996, a similar Forum of European National Nursing Associations and WHO was created, which shows every sign of becoming a very efficient channel for mobilizing the 4.5 million nurses and midwives in the Region for an HFA approach.

Collaborative networks are a recent development but they aim to be permanent international structures, with a tremendous potential for having a major influence on working towards specific HFA targets across the Region. As already mentioned, these include Regions for health, Healthy Cities, Health Promoting Schools and Health Promoting Hospitals, Health in Prisons, CINDI and, in a broader sense, the WHO Regional Committee. Other networks have been created to focus on the management of specific health problems, such as infectious diseases, (where specific task forces on STD/AIDS and on vaccination programmes in NIS have proved very effective in bringing many partners together), diabetes (the St Vincent movement) and stroke; several European cancer networks and the work of the International Agency for Research on Cancer (IARC) are also important in this connection.

> **NEHAPs – A PRACTICAL WAY OF BRINGING PARTNERS TOGETHER FOR ACTION**
>
> At the Second European Conference on Environment and Health (Helsinki, June 1994), ministers of health and the environment committed their respective countries to develop national environment and health action plans (NEHAPs) that explicitly link actions to improve the environment with the health of the population. Since then, 40 countries have completed or are in the process of developing their own NEHAPs. The NEHAPs have proved to be a successful mechanism for bringing various sectors and partners together and provide a coherent, comprehensive and cost-effective framework for action towards achieving HFA and the Agenda 21 goals. Because of the intersectoral nature of environment and health issues, successful and sustained implementation of NEHAPs is dependent on collaboration between all actors concerned at national and international levels, e.g. national governments, local authorities, different sectors of the economy and the public. Activities at country level are supported by international organizations and financial institutions. Also, the implementation of NEHAPs is used by a number of countries as part of their accession process to the European Union.
>
> Source: *Implementing national environmental health action plans in partnership*. Copenhagen, WHO Regional Office for Europe, 1999 (document submitted to the Third Ministerial Conference on Environment and Health, London, 1999).

While good progress has been made regarding the environment and health (through the NEHAP process), there is now an urgent need to create a new, strong Europe-wide movement for healthier lifestyles. The timing for this is right, and the technical knowledge and experience are available. The European Commission has developed a new health promotion action programme and the WHO Regional Office has widespread, strong networks and long experience in this field, as have many very active NGOs. Finally, and most importantly, there seems to be a growing political will in Member States to take the health promotion issue seriously.

Networks have tremendous potential for facilitating the exchange of knowledge and experience; other possible health-oriented networks of this type include parliamentary health committees and international associations of teachers, economists, lawyers, engineers and architects.

7.4 Planning, implementing and evaluating HFA policies

Making a reality of all the intentions outlined in Chapters 1–6 means nothing less than creating a broad societal movement for health involving the whole of civil, administrative, commercial and political society. This can be achieved only if all partners participate in the processes of understanding health problems and what is needed to achieve health improvement. For such broad processes to be effective, it is essential to have an inspiring vision of where to go, a transparent and mutually derived policy based on the HFA framework.

Starting in 1984, a large number of Member States in the European Region have moved ahead in adapting the regional HFA policy to their own needs. There was a temporary slow-down in the early 1990s, as political change and economic crisis in the CCEE and NIS brought short-term emergency health care reform to the centre stage. However, by June 1996, some 60% of the 51 countries currently making up the Region had formulated, or were developing, comprehensive policies for health based on the HFA approach, while most of the remaining countries had important elements of HFA included in their policies.

Policies and mechanisms for managing change

The mechanisms for implementing and monitoring HFA policies have been well thought out and thus very effective in a number of countries. In others, however, they have been fragmented, which has severely affected their effectiveness and impact. There has been a rich variety of ways in which countries have implemented their HFA policies, many making extensive use of quantified targets, others preferring to rely on qualitative objectives. The more successful have been extremely innovative in securing broad participation in decision-making, while others have limited their approach to an expert-led process confined largely to the health sector. Many countries have had their policies legitimized by their parliaments, thus ensuring broad-based political support over the medium term – a very important point. By and large, in recent years countries have become better at formulating national HFA policies and targets, and planning for their effective implementation.

The common framework of HFA indicators, and the common timetable for evaluation of the global, regional and national HFA policies and for reassessment of their scope and content against agreed targets, has also provided a new transparency in many countries. This process of continuous and systematic learning from experience has also changed, in a fundamental way, the basis for the periodic updating of policies – in essence, it has introduced a scientific principle into public policy-making. This new policy and process has created a new sense of cohesion and solidarity between Member States in the Region and has provided a unique knowledge base for all countries to learn from and be inspired by.

Thus, while a number of countries now have well functioning HFA-oriented policies, others need to update theirs and some still have to mobilize the political will to start the whole HFA policy-making process.

TARGET 21 – POLICIES AND STRATEGIES FOR HEALTH FOR ALL

BY THE YEAR 2010, ALL MEMBER STATES SHOULD HAVE AND BE IMPLEMENTING POLICIES FOR HEALTH FOR ALL AT COUNTRY, REGIONAL AND LOCAL LEVELS, SUPPORTED BY APPROPRIATE INSTITUTIONAL INFRASTRUCTURES, MANAGERIAL PROCESSES AND INNOVATIVE LEADERSHIP.

In particular:

21.1 policies for health for all at country level should provide motivation and an inspirational, forward-looking framework for policies and action in regions, cities, and local communities and in settings such as schools, workplaces and homes;

21.2 structures and processes should be in place for health policy development at country and other levels that bring together a broad range of key partners – public and private – with agreed mandates for policy formulation, implementation, monitoring and evaluation;

21.3 short-, medium-, and longer-term policy objectives, targets, indicators and priorities should be formulated, as well as the strategies to achieve them, based on the values of health for all, and progress towards their achievement should be regularly monitored and evaluated.

PROPOSED STRATEGIES

All Member States of the Region should ensure that their health policies are broadly in line with the HFA principles and strategies, so as to adapt their approaches to the health development needs and particular characteristics of today's democratic and pluralistic societies. Not only does this mean adapting the strategies outlined in Chapters 2–6 for dealing with lifestyles, environment and health issues; no less important is to embrace the concept of partnerships for planning and implementation, focused on the major settings/levels where action should take place. The HFA strategies and targets at European regional level should inspire those at country level, and country-level targets in turn should inspire the formulation of local targets. Some of the lessons that have been learned since 1984 are set out in the following pages.

7.4.1 Providing a clear map of the way forward

The actions which are needed to promote equity in health, strengthen sustainability and provide a sharper focus in health care call for long and determined efforts by many partners. Unless there is a written policy document which can be picked up, read, discussed, and even argued over, the many partners who must be involved will not clearly understand why they should work together for health, or what their particular input might be. An HFA policy document at country (and, when appropriate, subnational) and local levels – with clear objectives, strategies and targets – provides the essential framework, reference and starting point, so that even small incremental steps are made in the right direction. Creating such a map of the way forward requires a democratic, participatory, planning process, the essential steps of which are described below.

7.4.2 Creating awareness

Policy, actions and a commitment to health will not happen by themselves. It is an essential ongoing task of public health practitioners to create an awareness of the need to make health objectives part of society's overall socioeconomic development; in addition, the whole of the health sector must act as an advocate for health and for the promotion of equity and solidarity in health.

These processes entail understanding and providing a clearer picture of health experience and determinants, as well as of health inequities. Regular reports on these subjects at international, national, regional and local levels have an essential contribution to make here. Such reporting will not be successful if it is directed solely at the scientific community or health administrations; it must be designed to be understood by all prospective partners, focusing on politicians at all levels, as well as on professionals and the general public. Close cooperation with the media, and their constructive support, is therefore vital.

7.4.3 Agreeing on the process

As mentioned above, the policy development process must be transparent and ensure as broad a participation as possible by different sectors, levels, and interest groups. Unless those who are to carry out health and development policies and programmes also take part in their formulation and evaluation, they will feel little commitment to putting them into practice.

Agreement on a policy development process should include moves to create or strengthen mechanisms and infrastructures that facilitate cooperation among all major partners. Thus at country level, a special national health council could unite the leadership of health and other ministries, national employers' and employees' organizations, key national associations of health personnel, a national umbrella organization of local councils, and NGOs. Similar mechanisms (including, where relevant, subnational structures) would be needed at city/local community levels, with committees having a similar purpose at workplaces, schools and other institutions. All these mechanisms must deal with possible conflicts of interest, recognize the need for negotiation and compromise, and empower vulnerable groups to make their voices heard. At all levels, such committees need strong support from public health experts and input from different expert groups.

7.4.4 Searching for consensus

The essential basis for policy development at all levels is the achievement of a common understanding of underlying values, goals and objectives, and of the priorities to be assigned to them. This includes considering the weight to be given to the various values, defining the criteria for setting priorities, and discussing the possible consequences of various options. These processes will certainly involve negotiation and re-negotiation between the partners for health on a continuous basis, as the policy unfolds.

Changes in government at national, regional and local levels can make it difficult to secure commitment to long-term policies for health, which may not produce results until beyond the electoral cycle. However, it is easier to achieve long-term cross-party commitment when politicians at national, regional, city and local levels are involved at an early stage. Building a strong base of consumer or public support can also help to impart the necessary continuity and sustainability to policies for health.

7.4.5 Setting targets

The experience of the past 12 years in using the regional HFA targets and their indicators across Europe, as well as targets at national and local levels in many countries, has already proved that target-setting is a particularly valuable tool. Targets make policy objectives more specific, allow progress towards them to be monitored and inspire many partners to actively support health developments. In the ambitious approach to policy development proposed for the coming years, the use of targets at international, country and local levels will continue to be of great importance. The main reasons are:

- setting targets requires an assessment of the present situation to be made on as scientific a basis as possible, and some indication of possible future trends as an essential element in determining priorities;

- setting targets and monitoring progress towards them represents a vital learning experience in the continuing policy-making process, since it can focus discussion on what it had been hoped to achieve and why, and whether or not this was successful, and why;
- targets provide a powerful communication tool, taking policy-making out of bureaucratic confines and making it a clearly understood public issue;
- targets act as points on a map to give all partners a clearer understanding of the scope of the policy, why certain things must happen, and what might be their role in making them happen; they can also become a rallying point for groups at grassroots level to mobilize for, and demand, action;
- targets, monitored by specific indicators, are an excellent tool for strengthening accountability for health;
- in the short term, targets provide a reference point for assessing the advisability of day-to-day actions, i.e. evaluating proposals from government departments, or the annual budget;
- finally, by involving them in the actual process of target-setting, a major strategy has been created to motivate people for action.

Not all targets need to be quantified, and it is important to avoid the well known bias towards the easily measurable in target-setting. In setting targets, policy-makers must carefully consider the expected effectiveness of the proposed solutions and the possible implications of action, or inaction. As a minimum, targets should indicate aspirations for improved health and reductions in risk factors for health. It may also be helpful to set process targets that specify action levels at given points in time.

The main strategies by which targets might be reached should be outlined, showing how the major partners can contribute. Target-setting should also include a clear agreement as to when policy targets should be evaluated and updated; this is likely to be at least every ten years.

7.4.6 Achieving transparency

Whichever way is chosen for formulating objectives and targets, these must be expressed in a clear and transparent manner in the written policy and strategy document. It is this written form that allows the many partners involved to see what they have jointly committed themselves to achieving, and to understand their own potential role. To foster such understanding, different versions can be prepared for different target groups, and use can be made of new forms of dissemination such as the World Wide Web.

7.4.7 Legitimizing the process

The policy development process can be legitimized by means of a broad, transparent consultation process. Many excellent examples now exist from the work done since 1984 at national, regional and city levels of the positive contribution from public meetings, "road-shows", the mass media, and provision of feedback on the consultation process. Formal approval of the policy does need to be guaranteed at the highest political level, preferably by national or local parliaments, county or city councils. Without such high-level approval, the health sector will not have the influence needed to carry the policy through, working sometimes alone but very often with many other sectors and partners.

7.4.8 Creating new alliances

Forming new partnerships. The formulation and implementation of this type of policy requires not only the creation of new alliances with different sectors and with the many public and private partners involved, including a myriad of voluntary organizations, but also a different approach to building partnerships with these bodies.

Public health practitioners and the health sector must take primary responsibility for encouraging these other sectors and bodies to put health high on their agendas, and they will need strengthening in order to meet this challenge. Working together towards shared goals of health improvement will require new structures for involving all partners in health development. In building alliances with other sectors, there must be a search for common or converging objectives. The health sector should be ready to conduct a well documented and transparent dialogue, and to seek a balance or trade-offs when there appear to be conflicting objectives.

All this means learning not only about each other but also from each other. Most importantly, in seeking out, building up and carrying through partnerships, the creation and maintenance of a climate of trust will be vital. Strong but shared leadership, and effective organizational development, lie at the heart of successful partnerships for health. There must also be agreement on responsibilities, mechanisms and budgets, and an agreed basis for accountability.

7.4.9 Broadening the range of instruments for policy implementation

The action which may be taken to implement a policy may differ according to the level of responsibility and the existing policy environment. Certain laws or regulations can only be passed at the national level, or the regional level in federal countries. In the past, the tendency in relation to multisectoral action, for example, has been to concentrate on legislative and regulatory measures, and to a limited extent on financial measures, but more use should now be made of administrative, financial and management instruments, and of measures to affect research and training. The further use of health impact assessments and health policy audits will be essential.

Much more thought should also now be given to mechanisms to inform, involve and promote the rich networks of influence and development within civil societies. It is here, at a decentralized level within societies, that much of the commitment to and activities for health will actually occur.

7.4.10 Coordinating, monitoring and evaluating progress

Accountability can be achieved through mechanisms for coordinating, monitoring and evaluating progress in policy implementation and through procedures for reporting to elected bodies, as well as through the mass media. There are many good examples of such public health reporting, which allows for learning from experience, making the necessary adjustments and revisions to keep on track and to meet changing circumstances and conditions. Provision for this should be made in the HFA policy itself, which should also include precise indicators to measure progress towards each target, a clear mechanism for their collection and analysis and, finally, predetermined periods for evaluation timed to feed into the next planning cycle.

HFA POLICY DEVELOPMENT IN FINLAND – A CONTINUOUS PROCESS OF IMPLEMENTATION, EVALUATION AND REVISION

In 1985, the Finnish Government submitted to parliament, for discussion, a national HFA document with 32 policy statements. This was the first of its kind in Europe, and it was quickly followed by a strategy for its implementation. The implementation process did not run as smoothly as had been anticipated. Despite broad political consensus on the main policy directions, little attempt had been made to define priorities or assign responsibility for action. By 1990, it was decided to revise the policy and to combine this with an external review of the whole process (by WHO). The review process aroused considerable interest, since in the meantime the policy environment had changed; the economy was showing signs of depression; and a major reform of planning and financing was under way which entailed transferring responsibility for financing health services to the 455 municipalities.

The WHO review group noted that the policy process had been largely expert-led and confined to the health sector. Early involvement of other sectors and wider consultation processes, it was suggested, might have helped with implementation of the policy; the policy had not received high enough visibility in the mass media or at grassroots level; more specific objectives and targets for vulnerable groups might have increased the potential for promoting equity in health; and more human and financial resources should have been used for implementation and monitoring of the policy.

Following wide-ranging consultations, a revised strategy was approved in late 1992. The revised policy was more selective, specified the roles and tasks of all partners, and established a defined time frame. Much more emphasis was given to publicity, training and teaching materials. At the beginning of 1998, a new process of evaluation and revision was initiated. The new policy will have a two-year preparatory period which will involve widespread consultations with other groups and sectors. Particular attention is to be paid to future health challenges, the lifespan concept, and equity issues.

As the case of Finland clearly demonstrates, HFA is not a one-off measure but a continuous process of implementation, evaluation, and revision.

Sources: Health for all policy in Finland. WHO health policy review. Copenhagen, WHO Regional Office for Europe, 1991 (document EUR/FIN/HSC 410); *Exploring the process of health policy development in Europe.* Copenhagen, WHO Regional Office for Europe (in press).

Chapter 8

HEALTH21 – a new opportunity for action

As we enter the twenty-first century, the people of Europe are looking for change, for more purpose and fulfilment in their lives, and for more social responsibility. There will always be trade-offs between economic development and the protection and improvement of health, but there is a widely shared feeling that the current system is weighted too heavily in favour of economic gain. The two are intrinsically linked, yet the connection is often ignored. This neglect has got to change.

Health is unique; health is the flesh and bone of human development; it is both the precondition for a state of wellbeing and a prerequisite for the satisfaction of other needs. It concerns every individual and is easily understood by every member of society; health is everybody's business, and everyone must be involved in actions to improve it. Private and public sectors, professionals, NGOs, political leaders and others must be rallied around a common agenda – that is the democratic way.

Momentous opportunities are now within our grasp for improving the health of all the people of Europe. Much has been learned from successful initiatives developed in the health sector and in many other sectors, by many different actors, during the past 10–15 years. That is the good news; the bad news is that they often tend to remain isolated events. This tendency has got to change.

However, new "strategic approaches" in Europe are not enough; leadership is the key. Leadership that will recognize the formidable potential which health development has, not just to improve people's health but to strengthen social cohesion and purpose – i.e. to create a healthy society.

We need public health leaders who are willing to learn, by careful analysis of their own past experience and that of other countries. Leaders who will make future learning possible, too, by setting targets and measuring progress towards them; leaders who will facilitate good practice in a systematic way throughout their countries, and set an example to others.

Europe is uniquely positioned to provide such global leadership: it is a region where solidarity is an honourable word, a region with unparalleled collective knowledge, tools and technologies to promote health effectively.

Paradoxically, for a multitude of reasons, many European societies seem to be adrift. The political and religious certainties of the past have given way to a consumer society driven by technology and the imperative of profit. Many people are increasingly isolated and interact less with the society around them. In essence, they lack the basic human requirement for quality of life: to feel wanted and needed. This drift has got to change.

HEALTH21 offers a new opportunity for a sense of social purpose. Without such a framework, policy-makers at all levels and in all sectors can easily "lose sight of the wood for the trees", bending to vested interests and political factors. When that happens, their choices may not reflect the clear values and the true needs of their populations, and all too often their decisions will result in a worsening of health and greater costs to society as a whole.

This new HFA framework provides a mechanism for sorting out the tough decisions, for making appropriate allocations of resources, for encouraging all those whose actions create health, and for challenging those whose actions damage people's health. This approach is available for all to use; it is not the property of any one organization or sector. The general ideas must, however, be adapted to the wide range of different political, economic, social and cultural environments prevailing in the vast territory covered by the 51 Member States of the Region.

Making these changes for health will require leaders who can listen. They must listen to the voices of the people and their local concerns, to the views of health care providers and their technical expertise, and to the opinions of the many partners in the private and public sectors who contribute to the creation of population health.

People throughout Europe must feel that their health is secure. They must have the security of knowing that they have access throughout their lives to health care that is affordable, relevant, and of good quality. Health security encompasses the basic human right of every individual to a good standard of physical and mental health, including the right to sufficient, healthy food, the right to decent housing, the right to live and work in safe environments, and the right of access to education and information on health.

Sadly, in many countries and local communities, health does not receive anything like the attention and resources that are needed. It will take innovative changes in the way that societies do business to unlock the money, the human energy and the initiative to improve people's health. These resources must be unlocked.

Never before has Europe been confronted with such a promising potential for the future, but never before has the challenge to create effective yet inspiring governance been so great. The HFA movement in the European Region responds to this need. While health is everybody's business, public health leaders must now take charge and lead by ideas, inspiration and initiative. Public health leadership must lift health to the top of the political agenda, mobilize the tremendous resources of the European Region, and create a coalition of committed and compassionate men and women and organizations and countries with a unity of purpose. Such an achievement would echo around the world.

So we end this strategy, not with a conclusion, but with a call: an invitation to Europe's people, professions, organizations, institutions, and countries to embrace the HFA approach. We urge them to build policies upon its values, to take action to implement them, to share their measured outcomes and to learn from each other. Given the HFA framework to serve as the inspirational basis for pooling our collective enthusiasm and potential, we firmly believe that the year 2000 will truly be the start of a better future for the 51 Member States and the 870 million people of the European Region.

Annex 1

Relationship between global and regional HFA targets

HEALTH21 – HFA policy framework for the WHO European Region – 21 targets	Strategies for target attainment (highlights only)	HFA in the 21st century – 10 global targets
1. Solidarity for health in the European Region	Sharing of vision, resources, knowledge and expertise in Europe More and better coordinated external support to countries in need, in line with their HFA-based development plans	1. Increase equity in health
2. Equity in health	Reduction of social and economic inequities between groups, through policies, legislation and action	
3. Healthy start in life	Investment in social and economic wellbeing of parents and families Access to good reproductive and child health services	2. Improve survival and quality of life
4. Health of young people	Creation of supportive and safe physical, social and economic environments Cooperation of health, education and social services	
5. Healthy aging	Housing, income and other measures to enhance autonomy and social productivity Health promotion and protection throughout life	
6. Improving mental health	Living and working conditions shaped to gain a sense of coherence and social relations Quality services for people with mental health problems	3. Reverse global trends of five major pandemics

HEALTH21 – HFA policy framework for the WHO European Region – 21 targets	Strategies for target attainment (highlights only)	HFA in the 21st century – 10 global targets
7. Reducing communicable diseases	Eradication/elimination of poliomyelitis, measles and neonatal tetanus Internationally agreed surveillance, immunization and control strategies	4. Eradicate and eliminate certain diseases
8. Reducing noncommunicable diseases	Prevention and control of common noncommunicable disease risk factors Healthy public policies, including a Europe-wide movement for healthy lifestyles	3. Reverse global trends of five major pandemics
9. Reducing injury from violence and accidents	Higher priority to safety and social cohesion in living and working environments	
10. A healthy and safe physical environment	National and subnational action plans on environment and health Legal and economic instruments to reduce waste and pollution	5. Improve access to water, sanitation, food and shelter
11. Healthier living	Actions to facilitate healthy choices regarding nutrition, physical exercise and sexuality	6. Promote healthy lifestyles and discourage health-damaging ones
12. Reducing harm from alcohol, drugs and tobacco	Broad strategies to prevent addictions and treat victims	
13. Settings for health	Multisectoral mechanisms to make homes, schools, workplaces and cities more healthy	
14. Multisectoral responsibility for health	Through health impact assessment, all sectors to be accountable for their effects on health	
15. An integrated health sector	Primary health care for families and communities, with flexible systems of hospital referral	8. Improve access to comprehensive, essential, high-quality health care
16. Managing for quality of care	Health outcomes to drive health development programmes and patient care	

HEALTH21 – HFA policy framework for the WHO European Region – 21 targets	Strategies for target attainment (highlights only)	HFA in the 21st century – 10 global targets
17. Funding health services and allocating resources	Funding systems fostering universal coverage, solidarity and sustainability Sufficient financial resources allocated to priority health needs	
18. Developing human resources for health	Education based on HFA principles Public health professionals educated to act as key enablers and advocates for health from community to country level	
19. Research and knowledge for health	Orientation of research policies to HFA needs Mechanisms to base practice on scientific evidence	10. Support research for health 9. Implement global and national health information and surveillance systems
20. Mobilizing partners for health	Advocacy, coalition-building and joint action for health Sectors and actors identify and account for mutual benefits of investment in health	7. Develop, implement and monitor national HFA policies
21. Policies and strategies for health for all	HFA policies (with targets and indicators) formulated and implemented from country to community level, involving relevant sectors and organizations	

Annex 2

21 targets for the 21st century and suggested areas for formulating indicators

The experience gained since the 1980s of formulating HFA policies, and of monitoring and evaluating their implementation, together with feedback information from countries indicate the need for the regional targets to be realistic and achievable without being prescriptive. At the same time, the targets need to provide a challenge and an inspiration – "a blend of today's realities and tomorrow's dreams".

In general, the suggested target levels refer to WHO's European Region as a whole. However, the targets should not be taken as being equally applicable to all individual countries in the Region (except for the targets for the eradication and elimination of certain diseases, for example). In some cases, several countries may already have achieved the target level, and the target would therefore no longer be challenging for them; or the target level may be too ambitious for a few countries and not appear to be immediately realistic and achievable.

The suggested targets are not a prescriptive list: they are meant to inspire countries to set their own country-specific targets. As the formulation of targets needs to be sensitive to the levels of health status and other factors in different parts of the Region, countries are encouraged – where appropriate – to adjust and implement policies and targets according to their own circumstances.

In selecting indicators to monitor progress towards the regional targets, consideration has been given to ensuring as much continuity as possible with the previous HFA indicators. The majority of indicators are based on routinely collected health-related statistics or otherwise available data at national and international levels.

Target-setting

In formulating targets, consideration has been given to the importance of the problem, the nature or type of the target (e.g. quantitative, qualitative, outcome, process, input), the level at which the target should be attained (e.g. European, national, regional, local, programme), and the feasibility of attainment for Member States.

Quantitative target levels for the European Region have been set using projections based on historical trends and analysis of the current situation, subject to the availability and quality of data. Quantitative targets in general refer to regional averages and are of two types:

- achievement of a certain absolute level; or
- achievement of a certain percentage increase/decrease in the appropriate indicator.

The following general assumptions were made when outlining projections and setting target levels: countries which had recorded good progress in the past were expected to continue in the same or better way; countries with downward trends or presently in a bad situation were expected to start making progress at the average speed experienced by countries which had made good progress in the past. The feasibility of projected target levels was checked against present achievements in countries; in other words, it was assumed that the current best level achieved by a certain country in the Region or globally can be achieved in future by other countries as well.

Baseline and target dates

The baseline for those targets that are formulated as a percentage increase or decrease in a certain indicator is 1995. However, the "end date" has been chosen according to the nature and type of target. In principle, the end date of 2020 has been used for health outcome targets (with earlier dates for eradication or elimination of some diseases), while other types of targets have earlier dates.

Indicators for monitoring progress towards targets

The principle of "a blend of today's realities and tomorrow's dreams" also applies to the selection of indicators to monitor progress towards the regional targets. The majority of indicators remain the same and to a large extent are already included in countries' routine data collection systems. However, they should also include important indicators for which the availability and quality of data still have to be improved in European countries. At its forty-ninth session in September 1999, the WHO Regional Committee for Europe will approve the new list of indicators – until then the current set of indicators remains valid. The final list will be published in the European Health for All Series at the end of 1999. This annex therefore includes only a preliminary outline of areas where indicators may be set.

The same indicator (e.g. maternal mortality) may be relevant to more than one target. Statistical indicators are not applicable to all targets. In these cases, progress towards achieving the target will need to be evaluated from a qualitative description of the situation, the actions taken and the outcomes achieved.

Most indicators will be measured by means of routine registration systems. However, some important indicators will need to be measured or supplemented by population surveys; this can be facilitated by participating in the WHO/EURO project on health interview surveys (EUROHIS).

Data on the indicators should be disaggregated by age, gender and identifiable socioeconomic subgroups (as relevant and appropriate), to stimulate analysis of equity in health at country level and in the Region as a whole.

TARGET 1 – SOLIDARITY FOR HEALTH IN THE EUROPEAN REGION

> BY THE YEAR 2020, THE PRESENT GAP IN HEALTH STATUS BETWEEN MEMBER STATES OF THE EUROPEAN REGION SHOULD BE REDUCED BY AT LEAST ONE THIRD.

In particular:

1.1 the gap in life expectancy between the third of European countries with the highest and the third of countries with the lowest life expectancy levels should be reduced by at least 30%;

1.2 the range of values for major indicators of morbidity, disability and mortality among groups of countries should be reduced through accelerated improvement of the situation in those that are disadvantaged.

This target can be achieved if:

- *all countries contribute to reducing health gaps through international solidarity, mutual support and the sharing of resources, knowledge, information and experience, approaches that are essential for the future of Europe;*

- *all countries elaborate a comprehensive development plan directly linked to their policy for health for all and the common health vision for Europe;*

- *external support provided by countries, agencies and organizations is coordinated and directly relevant to the health and development plans formulated by the receiving country;*

- *international institutions and funding agencies, together with WHO, coordinate their action in health and health-related fields in order to increase the volume, synergy and effectiveness of their support to countries most in need in the Region;*

- *all countries ensure that socioeconomic, environmental and trade policies are not detrimental to health in other countries, and that they contribute as much as possible to the development of disadvantaged countries.*

Suggested areas for formulating indicators

- Mortality-based indicators (e.g. life expectancy) and age-standardized mortality rates (e.g. maternal mortality)
- Selected measurements of the incidence and prevalence of disability and morbidity
- Estimates of health expenditures and external assistance, whenever such information is available

TARGET 2 – EQUITY IN HEALTH

> BY THE YEAR 2020, THE HEALTH GAP BETWEEN SOCIOECONOMIC GROUPS WITHIN COUNTRIES SHOULD BE REDUCED BY AT LEAST ONE FOURTH IN ALL MEMBER STATES, BY SUBSTANTIALLY IMPROVING THE LEVEL OF HEALTH OF DISADVANTAGED GROUPS.

In particular:

2.1 the gap in life expectancy between socioeconomic groups should be reduced by at least 25%;

2.2 the values for major indicators of morbidity, disability and mortality in groups across the socioeconomic gradient should be more equitably distributed;

2.3 socioeconomic conditions that produce adverse health effects, notably differences in income, educational achievement and access to the labour market, should be substantially improved;

2.4 the proportion of the population living in poverty should be greatly reduced;

2.5 people having special needs as a result of their health, social or economic circumstances should be protected from exclusion and given easy access to appropriate care.

This target can be achieved if:

- *public policies are assessed with regard to their impact on equity, are gender-sensitive and give higher priority to disadvantaged groups in terms of income, services and social security;*
- *policies, including fiscal policies, ensure that access to educational and other social services does not depend on income;*
- *policies and legislation are aimed at implementing United Nations provisions on human rights, including those concerning women and children, and specific agreements and regulations on the rights of people with disabilities, migrants and refugees;*
- *all sectors in society assume their share of responsibility for reducing social and economic inequities and alleviating their consequences on health;*
- *public, private and voluntary resources are available to meet the social and health needs of the most vulnerable groups in society and provide access to appropriate, acceptable and sustainable care for all who need it;*
- *Member States improve and harmonize their health information systems to record important socioeconomic variables and analyse their relation to health conditions.*

Suggested areas for formulating indicators

- Main socioeconomic measurements (e.g. educational levels, unemployment, income)
- Differences in broad health status between identifiable socioeconomic groups and genders (e.g. (maternal) mortality, morbidity, disability and access to health care)

TARGET 3 – HEALTHY START IN LIFE

> BY THE YEAR 2020, ALL NEWBORN BABIES, INFANTS AND PRE-SCHOOL CHILDREN IN THE REGION SHOULD HAVE BETTER HEALTH, ENSURING A HEALTHY START IN LIFE.

In particular:

3.1 all Member States should ensure improvements in access to appropriate reproductive health, antenatal, perinatal and child health services;

3.2 the infant mortality rate should not exceed 20 per 1000 live births in any country; countries with rates currently below 20 per 1000 should strive to reach 10 or below;

3.3 countries with rates currently below 10 per 1000 should increase the proportion of newborn babies free from congenital disease or disability;

3.4 mortality and disability from accidents and violence in under 5-year-olds should be reduced by at least 50%;

3.5 the proportion of children born weighing less than 2500 g should be reduced by at least 20%, and the differences between countries should be significantly reduced.

This target can be achieved if:

- *Member States invest in the social and economic wellbeing of parents and families and implement policies that create a supportive family with wanted children and good parenting abilities, to ensure a healthy start in life for all children;*
- *Member States have a comprehensive policy and local community programmes to ensure appropriate services for family planning and reproductive health;*
- *women's health is given high priority in national and subnational policies;*
- *integrated primary health care services include a broad network of family planning services, perinatal health care based on essential technologies, promotion of child health, prevention of childhood diseases – including immunization of at least 95% of infants and young children – and appropriate treatment of sick children;*

- *public policies, social environments and health services encourage and support mothers to breastfeed, so that at least 60% of newborn babies are breastfed for the first six months of life;*
- *community action supported by legal instruments aims at drastically reducing the number of children who are abused, battered, abandoned or marginalized;*
- *parents have the means and skills to bring their children up and care for them in a social environment that protects the rights of the child;*
- *community authorities support families by ensuring a safe nurturing environment and health-promoting child care facilities;*
- *sectors dealing with education, health and welfare work jointly to support the development of infants and young children at times of family crisis;*
- *efforts are made to inform the public about developments in genetic technology, the options offered by such developments and their ethical implications.*

Suggested areas for formulating indicators

- Mortality indicators related to age groups and causes of death (e.g. perinatal, infant, maternal mortality)
- Selected measurements of health status and wellbeing of neonates and infants (e.g. birth weight, congenital diseases, nutrition, immunization)

TARGET 4 – HEALTH OF YOUNG PEOPLE[19]

> BY THE YEAR 2020, YOUNG PEOPLE IN THE REGION SHOULD BE HEALTHIER AND BETTER ABLE TO FULFIL THEIR ROLES IN SOCIETY.

In particular:

4.1 children and adolescents should have better life skills and the capacity to make healthy choices;

4.2 mortality and disability from violence and accidents[20] involving young people should be reduced by at least 50%;

4.3 the proportion of young people engaging in harmful forms of behaviour[21] such as drug, tobacco, and alcohol consumption should be substantially reduced;

4.4 the incidence of teenage pregnancies should be reduced by at least one third.

---

[19] Up to 18 years of age.
[20] See also target 9, "Reducing injury from violence and accidents".
[21] See also target 12, "Reducing harm from alcohol, drugs and tobacco".

This target can be achieved if:

- *Member States establish appropriate measures and structures to protect children as vulnerable members of society, as stated in the United Nations Convention on the Rights of the Child;*
- *public policies ensure the creation of supportive and safe physical, social and economic environments, making healthy choices the easy choices;*
- *all public sector policy decisions are reviewed to estimate their impact on the health of children and adolescents, their families and carers;*
- *education and employment policies facilitate the access of young people to an optimal level of education and to the labour market;*
- *health, education and social services work together to counter the causes of poor self-image among young people, enhance their capacity to cope with stressful life events and to build and maintain social relations, respond to their psychosocial requirements, and reach out to marginalized young people;*
- *Member States ensure access to measures to avoid unplanned parenthood, including information and support to young people;*
- *relevant research and evaluation tools are used to assess regularly the health status of children and adolescents, including their emotional health.*

Suggested areas for formulating indicators

- Mortality indicators related to appropriate age groups and causes of death
- Indicators on lifestyles of young people (e.g. smoking, alcohol, drugs, sexual behaviour)

TARGET 5 – HEALTHY AGING

BY THE YEAR 2020, PEOPLE OVER 65 YEARS SHOULD HAVE THE OPPORTUNITY OF ENJOYING THEIR FULL HEALTH POTENTIAL AND PLAYING AN ACTIVE SOCIAL ROLE.

In particular:

5.1 there should be an increase of at least 20% in life expectancy and in disability-free life expectancy at age 65 years;

5.2 there should be an increase of at least 50% in the proportion of people at age 80 years enjoying a level of health in a home environment that permits them to maintain autonomy, self-esteem and their place in society.

This target can be achieved if:

- *public policies including those related to housing, income and other measures that enhance people's autonomy and social productivity, take full account of the needs and views of older people;*
- *health policies prepare for healthy aging through health promotion and protection at earlier ages;*
- *health and social services at community level support the elderly in their everyday lives according to their needs and views, reach out to them and help them to become more active and to help themselves;*
- *each community develops programmes that coordinate, monitor and evaluate the services available to the elderly and ensures that sufficient resources are available for this task;*
- *policies allow older people to use the capacities remaining to them and provide access to appropriate care, outreach services, appliances and social support.*

Suggested areas for formulating indicators

- Mortality indicators related to appropriate age groups and causes of death
- Available statistics on morbidity and disability among the elderly

TARGET 6 – IMPROVING MENTAL HEALTH

BY THE YEAR 2020, PEOPLE'S PSYCHOSOCIAL WELLBEING SHOULD BE IMPROVED AND BETTER COMPREHENSIVE SERVICES SHOULD BE AVAILABLE TO AND ACCESSIBLE BY PEOPLE WITH MENTAL HEALTH PROBLEMS.

In particular:

6.1   the prevalence and adverse health impact of mental health problems should be substantially reduced and people should have an increased ability to cope with stressful life events;

6.2   suicide rates should be reduced by at least one third, with the most significant reductions achieved in countries and population groups with currently high rates.

This target can be achieved if:

- *more attention is paid to the promotion and protection of mental health throughout life, particularly in socially and economically disadvantaged groups;*

- *living and working environments are shaped to help people at all ages to gain a sense of coherence, build and maintain social relations, and cope with stressful situations and events;*
- *health and other caring professions are trained in the early detection of mental health problems and appropriate intervention;*
- *services for people with mental health problems provide care of good quality, with an appropriate blend of community-based and hospital-based services, paying particular attention to crisis intervention and to minorities and disadvantaged groups;*
- *human rights are respected and the quality of life is improved for people with mental health problems, particularly those with chronic disorders.*

Suggested areas for formulating indicators

- Suicide rate
- Incidence and prevalence of mental disorders such as schizophrenia, serious depression, alcoholic psychosis, post-traumatic mental sequelae
- Statistics on availability and use of mental health services

TARGET 7 – REDUCING COMMUNICABLE DISEASES

BY THE YEAR 2020, THE ADVERSE HEALTH EFFECTS OF COMMUNICABLE DISEASES SHOULD BE SUBSTANTIALLY DIMINISHED THROUGH SYSTEMATICALLY APPLIED PROGRAMMES TO ERADICATE, ELIMINATE OR CONTROL INFECTIOUS DISEASES OF PUBLIC HEALTH IMPORTANCE.

In particular:

Elimination of disease[22]

7.1 by 2000 or earlier, poliomyelitis transmission in the Region should stop, and by 2003 or earlier this should be certified in every country;

7.2 by 2005 or earlier, neonatal tetanus should be eliminated from the Region;

7.3 by 2007 or earlier, indigenous measles should be eliminated from the Region, and by 2010 the elimination should be certified in every country;

Control of disease

7.4 by 2010 or earlier, all countries should have:

---

[22] For definitions of "eradication", "elimination" and "control", see Glossary of terms (Annex 5).

- an incidence level for diphtheria of below 0.1 per 100 000 population;
- new hepatitis B virus carrier incidence reduced by at least 80% through integration of hepatitis B vaccine in the child immunization programme;
- an incidence level of below 1 per 100 000 population for mumps, pertussis and invasive disease caused by *Haemophilus influenzae* type b;
- an incidence level for congenital syphilis of below 0.01 per 1000 live births;
- an incidence level for congenital rubella of below 0.01 per 1000 live births;

7.5 by 2015 or earlier:
- malaria should in any country be reduced to an incidence level of below 5 per 100 000 population, and there should be no deaths from indigenously-acquired malaria in the Region;
- every country should show a sustained and continuing reduction in the incidence, mortality and adverse consequences of HIV infection and AIDS, other sexually transmitted diseases, tuberculosis, and acute respiratory and diarrhoeal diseases in children.

This target can be achieved if:
- *public health systems with effective laboratory-based disease surveillance monitor the target diseases and detect emerging diseases and changing antiobiotic resistance pattern without delay;*
- *95% coverage is achieved within the eligible population against diseases preventable by immunization and targeted for elimination or control;*
- *universal immunization is achieved in childhood against rubella, and locally appropriate immunization strategies against hepatitis B are implemented, as well as vaccination programmes against Haemophilus influenzae type b and mumps, including the use of combination vaccines;*
- *integrated and culturally sensitive programmes for information, prevention and treatment of HIV/AIDS and sexually transmitted diseases are established, focusing on drug users and other particularly vulnerable groups;*
- *internationally agreed disease prevention and control strategies, such as those for tuberculosis, acute respiratory infections and diarrhoeal diseases, are implemented;*
- *in all countries, efforts are made to strengthen capabilities in malaria surveillance and interventions for the prevention of transmission, case detection and treatment;*
- *national and international collaboration partners, including networks of public health institutes and WHO collaborating centres, engage in the rapid exchange of information to*

act on epidemics and to guide policies, international collaboration, and health recommendations for travel and trade;

- *properly defined national and international strategies for elimination and control are developed, and implemented through multisectoral approaches and a well organized public health service.*

Suggested areas for formulating indicators

- Mortality indicators related to appropriate age groups and infectious diseases (tuberculosis, respiratory and diarrhoeal diseases, malaria, etc.)
- New cases of selected communicable diseases, i.e. measles, malaria, diphtheria, tetanus, pertussis, congenital syphilis, congenital rubella, neonatal tetanus, rubella, mumps, tuberculosis, hepatitis (A, B, other), syphilis, gonorrhoea, HIV/AIDS
- Percentage of children immunized against selected communicable diseases, i.e. diphtheria, tetanus, pertussis, measles, poliomyelitis, tuberculosis, *Haemophilus influenzae* type b, hepatitis B, mumps, rubella

TARGET 8 – REDUCING NONCOMMUNICABLE DISEASES

> BY THE YEAR 2020, MORBIDITY, DISABILITY AND PREMATURE MORTALITY DUE TO MAJOR CHRONIC DISEASES SHOULD BE REDUCED TO THE LOWEST FEASIBLE LEVELS THROUGHOUT THE REGION.

In particular:

8.1 mortality due to cardiovascular diseases in people under 65 years should be reduced on average by at least 40%, particularly in countries with currently high mortality;

8.2 mortality due to cancers of all sites in people under 65 years should be reduced on average by at least 15%, with mortality due to lung cancer reduced by 25%;

8.3 the incidence of diabetes-related amputations, blindness, kidney failure, pregnancy complications and other serious health effects should be reduced by one third;

8.4 there should be a sustained and continuing reduction in morbidity, disability and mortality due to chronic respiratory diseases, musculoskeletal disorders and other prevalent chronic conditions;

8.5 at least 80% of children aged 6 years should be free of caries, and 12-year-old children should have on average no more than 1.5 decayed, missing or filled teeth.

This target can be achieved if:

- *healthy public policies in all Member States focus on the implementation of health promotion and disease prevention principles and strategies, with full community participation;*
- *the prevention and control of common risk factors of noncommunicable diseases is made an integral part of community life, and a strong Europe-wide movement for healthy lifestyles involves all countries and relevant international organizations;*
- *comprehensive disease management is provided, with emphasis on health outcome and development of the quality of care, taking into account the rights and wishes of the patient;*
- *Member States develop and implement strategies for oral health, including caries prevention.*

Suggested areas for formulating indicators

- Mortality from major noncommunicable diseases (cardiovascular diseases, cancer, chronic respiratory diseases, diabetes, others) by age group
- Incidence and prevalence of the major noncommunicable diseases listed above, including asthma and chronic rheumatic diseases
- Hospital discharge statistics on major noncommunicable diseases
- Prevalence of major risk factors in the population, i.e. elevated blood pressure and serum cholesterol, inadequate physical activity, smoking, inappropriate nutrition
- Selected indicators for oral health

TARGET 9 – REDUCING INJURY FROM VIOLENCE AND ACCIDENTS

> BY THE YEAR 2020, THERE SHOULD BE A SIGNIFICANT AND SUSTAINABLE DECREASE IN INJURIES, DISABILITY AND DEATH ARISING FROM ACCIDENTS AND VIOLENCE IN THE REGION.

In particular:

9.1 mortality and disability from road traffic accidents should be reduced by at least 30%;

9.2 mortality and disability from all work, domestic and leisure accidents should be reduced by at least 50%, with the largest reductions in countries with current high levels of mortality from accidents;

9.3 the incidence of and mortality from domestic, gender-related and organized violence and its health consequences should be reduced by at least 25%.

This target can be achieved if:

- *public policies give higher priority to issues related to social cohesion and safety in the living and working environments and address the major determinants of violence and accidents, paying particular attention to alcohol consumption;*
- *all sectors cooperate in action to prevent accidents and violence whenever possible, and assist in dealing with the consequences and costs to victims and their families and to society;*
- *appropriate and gender-sensitive support, care and rehabilitation services are accessible to all people concerned with violence;*
- *countries undertake and cooperate on research into the forms, determinants and consequences of violence and accidents, analyse their incidence and make plans for preventive action;*
- *countries establish clear policies and guidelines related to road safety and include information on road safety in school curricula.*

Suggested areas for formulating indicators

- Mortality from main external causes of injury and poisoning
- Incidence of injuries due to traffic, home and work-related accidents
- Estimates of injury-related disability

TARGET 10 – A HEALTHY AND SAFE PHYSICAL ENVIRONMENT

> BY THE YEAR 2015, PEOPLE IN THE REGION SHOULD LIVE IN A SAFER PHYSICAL ENVIRONMENT, WITH EXPOSURE TO CONTAMINANTS HAZARDOUS TO HEALTH AT LEVELS NOT EXCEEDING INTERNATIONALLY AGREED STANDARDS.

In particular:

10.1 population exposure to physical, microbial and chemical contaminants in water, air, waste and soil that are hazardous to health should be substantially reduced, according to the timetable and reduction rates stated in national environment and health action plans;

10.2 people should have universal access to sufficient quantities of drinking-water of a satisfactory quality.

This target can be achieved if:

- *national, regional and local action plans for preventing and reducing environmental health risks are developed and implemented, and suitable legal and economic instruments are used to reduce consumption, waste and pollution;*

- *air quality in urban areas is improved by reducing pollution originating from industrial, transport and household sources to meet WHO air quality guidelines;*
- *steps are taken to ensure supply to every home of drinking-water meeting WHO guidelines for water quality, and global water management practices including pollution control measures are strengthened;*
- *proper wastewater management systems are provided, including collection, treatment and final disposal or re-use of all waste waters;*
- *waste producers implement systems ensuring waste collection and treatment, including the enforcement of policies and structures for recycling and minimizing wastes;*
- *emergency response and capacity plans are developed for all nuclear power plants, and safety standards implemented, using the best available technology;*
- *international conventions such as those on transboundary waters, biological diversity, climate change, long-range transboundary air pollution, and protection of the ozone layer, are implemented;*
- *adequate capacities are built up for inspection and monitoring of health risks in the environment, and data collection and monitoring exercises on environmental contamination and health effects are undertaken on a regular basis and their results made freely accessible;*
- *public awareness of sustainable development and environmental protection is enhanced.*

Suggested areas for formulating indicators

- Percentage of population with adequate water supply in the home and hygienic sewage disposal
- Statistics on microbiological foodborne diseases – outbreaks and persons affected
- Statistics on the emission of selected pollutants

TARGET 11 – HEALTHIER LIVING[23]

> BY THE YEAR 2015, PEOPLE ACROSS SOCIETY SHOULD HAVE ADOPTED HEALTHIER PATTERNS OF LIVING.

In particular:

11.1 healthier behaviour in such fields as nutrition, physical activity, and sexuality should be substantially increased;

11.2 there should be a substantial increase in the availability, affordability and accessibility of safe and healthy food.

---

[23] For stress prevention, see target 6 "Improving mental health".

This target can be achieved if:

- *public policies place health at the centre of human development and facilitate healthy choices;*
- *people are enabled to develop and use their own potential in order to lead socially, economically and mentally fulfilling lives;*
- *principles of food hygiene are applied throughout the entire food chain from production to consumption, and all sectors share responsibility for their application;*
- *regulations to reduce microbial and chemical contamination of food are implemented, and international standards in animal husbandry and food hygiene are applied;*
- *the balance of nutrition is improved and vitamin and mineral deficiencies (such as vitamin A and iron) are eliminated, by increasing the availability of, access to and consumption of whole-grain cereals, pulses, vegetables and fruits and by reducing the consumption of high-fat food;*
- *iodine deficiency disorders[24] are eliminated as a public health problem in all countries, by implementing universal salt iodization strategies;*
- *fiscal, agricultural and retail policies to encourage healthier nutrition are implemented;*
- *transport, urban planning and settlement policies encourage recreation and increased physical activity;*
- *information on safer sex practices reaches all people;*
- *effective infrastructures and resources are provided to make existing knowledge about health better known, through appropriate education and information.*

Suggested areas for formulating indicators

- National statistics on food consumption and body mass index
- Available data on estimates of physical activity and sexual behaviour

---

[24] Resolution WHA49.13 (1997) reaffirms the goal of eliminating iodine deficiency disorders as a public health problem in all countries by the year 2000.

Target 12 – Reducing harm from alcohol, drugs and tobacco

> BY THE YEAR 2015, THE ADVERSE HEALTH EFFECTS FROM THE CONSUMPTION OF ADDICTIVE SUBSTANCES SUCH AS TOBACCO, ALCOHOL AND PSYCHOACTIVE DRUGS SHOULD HAVE BEEN SIGNIFICANTLY REDUCED IN ALL MEMBER STATES.

In particular:

12.1 in all countries, the proportion of nonsmokers should be at least 80%, in over 15-year-olds and close to 100% in under 15-year-olds[25];

12.2 in all countries, per capita alcohol consumption should not increase or exceed 6 litres per annum, and should be close to zero in under 15-year-olds;

12.3 in all countries, the prevalence of illicit psychoactive drug use should be reduced by at least 25% and mortality by at least 50%.

This target can be achieved if:

- *educational and intervention strategies aim at improving the life skills and psychosocial wellbeing of people, helping them to manage life situations and make healthy choices;*
- *regulatory practices to limit exposure to environmental tobacco smoke and reduce alcohol intoxication, including drinking and driving, are enforced;*
- *risk-containment strategies are implemented to reduce the harm done by drug use;*
- *internationally agreed conventions for illicit drugs are implemented, and an internationally agreed convention for tobacco products is developed;*
- *fiscal and regulatory policies are established to limit the availability, accessibility and marketing of tobacco and alcohol products, notably to young people, and a complete advertising ban is placed on tobacco in all countries;*
- *communication strategies aim at generating public support for reducing the harm from addictive substances.*

Suggested areas for formulating indicators

- Mortality from alcohol- and drug-related causes of death
- Estimates of smoking prevalence in appropriate population groups and national statistics on tobacco consumption
- Estimates of alcohol use prevalence and national statistics on alcohol consumption
- Hospital admission statistics in relation to alcoholic psychosis and drug treatment

---

[25] Or other age limits as appropriate to national legislation.

Target 13 – Settings for Health

> BY THE YEAR 2015, PEOPLE IN THE REGION SHOULD HAVE GREATER OPPORTUNITIES TO LIVE IN HEALTHY PHYSICAL AND SOCIAL ENVIRONMENTS AT HOME, AT SCHOOL, AT THE WORKPLACE AND IN THE LOCAL COMMUNITY.

In particular:

13.1 the safety and quality of the home environment should be improved, through increased personal and family skills for health promotion and protection, and the health risks from the physical home environment should be reduced;

13.2 people with disabilities should have substantially improved opportunities for health and access to home, work, public and social life in accordance with the United Nations Standard Rules on the Equalization of Opportunities for Persons with Disabilities;[26]

13.3 home and work accidents should be reduced as specified in target 10;

13.4 at least 50% of children should have the opportunity of being educated in a health-promoting kindergarten, and 95% in a health-promoting school;[27]

13.5 at least 50% of cities, urban areas and communities should be active members of a healthy city or healthy community network;

13.6 at least 10% of medium- and large-sized companies should commit themselves to practising healthy company/enterprise principles.[28]

This target can be achieved if:

- *mechanisms are set up to allow people to influence the design and improvement of their living and work environment, and to participate in promoting health and wellbeing in their community;*
- *social organizations play a decisive role in increasing social cohesion and improving access to community coping resources;*

---

[26] As contained in an annex to United Nations General Assembly resolution 48/96 of 20 December 1993.
[27] The health-promoting school includes education for health in the school curriculum and in the activities of school health services. A health-promoting schools network has been run jointly by WHO, the European Commission and the Council of Europe since 1992.
[28] Healthy company/enterprise principles include a safe working environment, healthy working practices, programmes to promote health and address psychosocial risk factors at the workplace, health impact assessment for marketed products, and contribution to health and social development in the community.

- *an effective infrastructure for environmental health protection is available in terms of drinking-water supply, wastewater treatment and wastewater disposal, building requirements and protection from risks in the home and in the city;*
- *all sectors concerned support the integration of health-related issues into a comprehensive approach that enables schools to promote the physical, social and emotional health of students, staff, families and communities;*
- *the process of creating healthier cities is encouraged and supported, with the participation of partners from the fields of health, the environment, the economy, ecology, education, town planning and urban management.*

Suggested areas for formulating indicators

- Incidence and mortality indicators related to home and work accidents and occupational diseases
- National housing statistics

TARGET 14 – MULTISECTORAL RESPONSIBILITY FOR HEALTH

> BY THE YEAR 2020, ALL SECTORS SHOULD HAVE RECOGNIZED AND ACCEPTED THEIR RESPONSIBILITY FOR HEALTH.

In particular:

14.1 decision-makers in all sectors should take into consideration the benefits to be gained from investing for health in their particular sector and orient policies and actions accordingly;

14.2 Member States should have established mechanisms for health impact assessment and ensured that all sectors become accountable for the effects of their policies and actions on health.

This target can be achieved if:

- *Member States establish incentives and take legal and managerial measures which facilitate sectoral involvement and intersectoral collaboration for health;*
- *the promotion and protection of public health are used as essential criteria when choosing policies and strategies, both in business and in the public sector;*
- *Member States, individually and in collaboration, strengthen the evidence base on the health implications of actions by different sectors;*

- *governments and parliaments give higher priority to policies that contribute to health promotion and protection, and undertake health audits across all sectors;*
- *public inquiries and hearings are organized on the health impact of major projects, and broad participation of the public is ensured in assessment and dissemination of results;*
- *more attention is paid to individual and collective responsibility in education, information and research activities, in order to build awareness of competence in and accountability for health.*

Suggested areas for formulating indicators

- No statistical indicators; qualitative assessment only

TARGET 15 – AN INTEGRATED HEALTH SECTOR

> BY THE YEAR 2010, PEOPLE IN THE REGION SHOULD HAVE MUCH BETTER ACCESS TO FAMILY- AND COMMUNITY-ORIENTED PRIMARY HEALTH CARE, SUPPORTED BY A FLEXIBLE AND RESPONSIVE HOSPITAL SYSTEM.

In particular:

15.1 at least 90% of countries should have comprehensive primary health care services, ensuring continuity of care through efficient and cost-effective systems of referral to, and feedback from, secondary and tertiary hospital services;

15.2 at least 90% of countries should have family health physicians and nurses working at the core of this integrated primary health care service, using multiprofessional teams from the health, social and other sectors and involving local communities;

15.3 at least 90% of countries should have health services that ensure individuals' participation and recognizes and supports people as producers of health care.

This target can be achieved if:

- *appropriate primary health care services and programmes are designed, with the participation of local communities, to respond to needs and expectations in health promotion, disease prevention, care and rehabilitation, including activities to reach out to groups with special needs;*
- *the management of health services respects the principle that whatever care can satisfactorily be provided at the primary level should be, while referrals to secondary and tertiary hospital care are limited to cases requiring specialist skills and facilities;*

- *policies are formulated that support people in preserving their own health and caring for themselves whenever they can, and mechanisms are established, and information provided, to enable people to make informed choices on health matters and participate in decision-making.*

Suggested areas for formulating indicators

- Health personnel resources (e.g. physicians by speciality, nurses, and proportion with occupation within primary health care or hospitals)
- Availability of hospital beds by type, and other statistics on health care resources
- Indicators of health care consumptions (e.g. hospital admissions, average length of stay, ambulatory care contacts)

TARGET 16 – MANAGING FOR QUALITY OF CARE

> BY THE YEAR 2010, MEMBER STATES SHOULD ENSURE THAT THE MANAGEMENT OF THE HEALTH SECTOR, FROM POPULATION-BASED HEALTH PROGRAMMES TO INDIVIDUAL PATIENT CARE AT THE CLINICAL LEVEL, IS ORIENTED TOWARDS HEALTH OUTCOMES.

In particular:

16.1 the effectiveness of major public health strategies should be assessed in terms of health outcomes, and decisions regarding alternative strategies for dealing with individual health problems should increasingly be taken by comparing health outcomes and their cost–effectiveness;

16.2 all countries should have a nationwide mechanism for continuous monitoring and development of the quality of care for at least ten major health conditions, including measurement of health impact, cost–effectiveness and patient satisfaction;

16.3 health outcomes in at least five of the above health conditions should show a significant improvement, and surveys should show an increase in patient's satisfaction with the quality of services received and heightened respect for their rights.

This target can be achieved if:

- *all establishments providing health care adopt practices based on scientifically validated evidence, both in routine care and when new procedures are introduced, with quality of care indicators defined at the level of clinical care, and monitoring of the quality of care becoming an integral part of the work of each care unit;*

- *Member States develop policies and mechanisms that guarantee the rights of patients, including respect of their moral, cultural, religious and philosophical values and convictions, and promote open public debate on the ethical aspects of health policy and health care;*
- *educational and other measures provide health care professionals with the motivation and skills necessary to adopt the best practices and to be accountable for the outcome of their work;*
- *health outcomes and cost–effectiveness criteria are regularly used when procedures and practices are evaluated;*
- *new and existing technologies, including pharmaceuticals, are continuously monitored and assessed with respect to health impact, outcome and cost–effectiveness;*
- *a system is established to document, monitor and improve outcomes of care, and routine documentation on outcomes is disseminated to care providers on an anonymous basis;*
- *information on evidence-based practice is readily available to health care providers.*

Suggested areas for formulating indicators

- Mortality from selected conditions (e.g. appendicitis, hernia, intestinal obstruction, adverse effects of therapeutic agents and other "avoidable" causes of death)
- Specific indicators related to the quality of health care (surgical wound infection rates, diabetic complications, autopsy rates, patients' satisfaction estimates, etc.)

TARGET 17 – FUNDING HEALTH SERVICES AND ALLOCATING RESOURCES

BY THE YEAR 2010, MEMBER STATES SHOULD HAVE SUSTAINABLE FINANCING AND RESOURCE ALLOCATION MECHANISMS FOR HEALTH CARE SYSTEMS BASED ON THE PRINCIPLES OF EQUAL ACCESS, COST–EFFECTIVENESS, SOLIDARITY, AND OPTIMUM QUALITY.

In particular:

17.1 spending on health services should be adequate, while corresponding to the health needs of the population;

17.2 resources should be allocated between health promotion and protection, treatment and care, taking account of health impact, cost–effectiveness and the available scientific evidence;

17.3 funding systems for health care guarantee universal coverage, solidarity and sustainability.

This target can be achieved if:

- *public health infrastructures are strengthened;*
- *health priorities are determined in a transparent fashion, and sufficient financial resources are allocated to defined priorities, aiming at optimizing health gains;*
- *health sector resources, where appropriate, are allocated to other sectors and to private and nongovernmental organizations, to pursue commonly defined health goals;*
- *measures aiming at containing costs are brought to bear primarily on health care establishments and providers, rather than on patients and users of services;*
- *mechanisms are established to monitor the effect of funding and resource allocation on health service delivery and the health of the population.*

Suggested areas for formulating indicators

- Health expenditures, total and by component (public, recurring hospital expenditures, capital investment, pharmaceuticals, etc.)

TARGET 18 – DEVELOPING HUMAN RESOURCES FOR HEALTH

> BY THE YEAR 2010, ALL MEMBER STATES SHOULD HAVE ENSURED THAT HEALTH PROFESSIONALS AND PROFESSIONALS IN OTHER SECTORS HAVE ACQUIRED APPROPRIATE KNOWLEDGE, ATTITUDES AND SKILLS TO PROTECT AND PROMOTE HEALTH.

In particular:

18.1 the education of health professionals should be based on the principles of the HFA policy, preparing them to provide promotive, preventive, curative and rehabilitative services of good quality and helping to bridge clinical and public health practice;

18.2 planning systems should be in place to ensure that the number and mix of health professionals trained meet current and future health needs;

18.3 all Member States should have adequate capacity for specialized training in public health leadership, management and practice;

18.4 the education of professionals in other sectors should include the basic principles of the HFA policy and, specifically, knowledge of how their work can influence the determinants of health.

This target can be achieved if:

- *all education of health professionals imparts the relevant knowledge, attitudes and skills for health care practice, including good quality public health practice, and the essential aspects of economics and social sciences relevant to attaining health for all;*
- *education programmes focused on family care are established in all educational institutions and universities where physicians, nurses and other health professionals are trained;*
- *the education of public health professionals prepares them to act as enablers, mediators and advocates for health in all sectors, and to work with a broad set of partners in society;*
- *the education of professionals in other sectors prepares them to recognize the importance and benefit of their policies and actions for population health;*
- *educational institutions have systems which ensure continuous feedback of experience from practice and use modern educational techniques and technologies.*

Suggested areas for formulating indicators

- Statistics on health personnel resources by category, as appropriate
- Statistics on medical professionals graduating

TARGET 19 – RESEARCH AND KNOWLEDGE FOR HEALTH

> BY THE YEAR 2005, ALL MEMBER STATES SHOULD HAVE HEALTH RESEARCH, INFORMATION AND COMMUNICATION SYSTEMS THAT BETTER SUPPORT THE ACQUISITION, EFFECTIVE UTILIZATION, AND DISSEMINATION OF KNOWLEDGE TO SUPPORT HEALTH FOR ALL.

In particular:

19.1 all countries should have research policies oriented towards the priorities of their long-term policies for health for all;

19.2 all countries should have mechanisms that enable health services delivery and development to be based on scientific evidence;

19.3 health information should be useful to and easily accessible by politicians, managers, health and other professionals, as well as the general public;

19.4 all countries should have established health communication policies and programmes which support the agenda of health for all and facilitate access to such information.

This target can be achieved if:

- *Member States formulate health research strategies based on the values of health for all, striking a balance between basic and applied research;*
- *international cooperation is strengthened, leading to an increase in the number of intercountry research programmes and better exchange of research information;*
- *the public sector strengthens communication and cooperation between the scientific community and decision-makers for the application of new knowledge to health development;*
- *health and health-related information bases are set up and maintained to support the monitoring and evaluation of health policies and programmes, enhance accountability for health, facilitate the sharing of knowledge within and between countries, and help raise people's health awareness;*
- *the resources and expertise of the media and communication sector are fully engaged to inform, educate and persuade all people of the individual and collective importance of health, and to give them options for action.*

Suggested areas for formulating indicators

- Expenditure on health research and development

TARGET 20 – MOBILIZING PARTNERS FOR HEALTH

> BY THE YEAR 2005, IMPLEMENTATION OF POLICIES FOR HEALTH FOR ALL SHOULD ENGAGE INDIVIDUALS, GROUPS AND ORGANIZATIONS THROUGHOUT THE PUBLIC AND PRIVATE SECTORS, AND CIVIL SOCIETY, IN ALLIANCES AND PARTNERSHIPS FOR HEALTH.

In particular:

20.1 the health sector should engage in active promotion and advocacy for health, encouraging other sectors to join in multisectoral activities and share goals and resources;

20.2 structures and processes should exist at international, country, regional and local levels to facilitate harmonized collaboration of all actors and sectors in health development.

This target can be achieved if:

- *existing partnerships for health and social development, such as the networks of cities, schools and workplaces, are strengthened and the potential for new partnerships at all levels is explored;*

- *all sectors and actors in health identify and take into account the mutual benefits of investment in health;*
- *mechanisms are in place to facilitate the joint development, implementation and evaluation of policies and strategies based on the principles of health for all;[29]*
- *health professionals are responsive to the motivations of professionals in other sectors and willing to negotiate for policies that are mutually beneficial;*
- *emphasis is placed at each level on building alliances and partnerships for health, empowering people and creating networks;*
- *public health leadership is provided which motivates, inspires, facilitates and engages all sectors for health;*
- *international solidarity for health development is strengthened, using the European structures for intergovernmental cooperation and action.*

Suggested areas for formulating indicators

- No statistical indicators; qualitative assessment only

TARGET 21 – POLICIES AND STRATEGIES FOR HEALTH FOR ALL

> BY THE YEAR 2010, ALL MEMBER STATES SHOULD HAVE AND BE IMPLEMENTING POLICIES FOR HEALTH FOR ALL AT COUNTRY, REGIONAL AND LOCAL LEVELS, SUPPORTED BY APPROPRIATE INSTITUTIONAL INFRASTRUCTURES, MANAGERIAL PROCESSES AND INNOVATIVE LEADERSHIP.

In particular:

21.1 policies for health for all at country level should provide motivation and an inspirational, forward-looking framework for policies and action in regions, cities, and local communities and in settings such as schools, workplaces and homes;

21.2 structures and processes should be in place for health policy development at country and other levels that bring together a broad range of key partners – public and private – with agreed mandates for policy formulation, implementation, monitoring and evaluation;

21.3 short-, medium-, and longer-term policy objectives, targets, indicators and priorities should be formulated, as well as the strategies to achieve them, based on the values of health for all, and progress towards their achievement should be regularly monitored and evaluated.

---

[29] See target 21, "Policies and strategies for health for all".

This target can be achieved if:

- *policies for health for all are endorsed by the highest political body at each level;*
- *public health infrastructures and functions are strengthened and modernized in line with public health needs and the values of health for all at country, regional and local levels;*
- *health status and trends[30] are regularly assessed, the health development process is monitored, and the impact of policies on health outcomes, health determinants and public satisfaction is evaluated;*
- *countries carry out periodic population-based surveys, based on WHO methodology;*
- *all countries have a harmonized, comparable data collection system for monitoring progress towards health for all, and greater efforts are made to streamline data collection and establish a more uniform selection of indicators, to ensure that health information and communication systems are internationally coordinated and harmonized;*
- *policies and strategies are formulated through the full mobilization of partners.[31]*

Suggested areas for formulating indicators

- No statistical indicators; qualitative assessment only

---

[30] Especially targets 1 to 9.
[31] See target 20, "Mobilizing partners for health".

Annex 3

Schedule of main events 1998–2005

Major events in monitoring, evaluation and implementation of the HFA policy for the WHO European Region

The HFA policy provides a visionary framework for health improvement in Europe. This schedule is complementary to other actions at national and local levels. It proposes a number of specific events in countries, as well as various major consultations or conferences to be organized by the Regional Office. The relevant statutory functions of the Regional Committee are likewise included.

It should be noted that a more detailed strategic plan of work by the Regional Office in support of implementation of the renewed HFA policy will be included in the biennial regional programme budgets for the period 2000–2005.

The aim of this schedule for the European Regional Organization of WHO is to promote an integrated partnership approach at local, regional, country and Europe-wide levels. The Regional Office will further strengthen its international activities through establishment of and participation in partnerships such as the Interagency Immunization Coordinating Committee (IICC), the International Task Force for Sexually Transmitted Disease Prevention and Control and the EEHC.

"HEALTH21" Chapter	Action to be taken by:			
	Year	Member States	Regional Committee	Regional Office
7	1998		Approval of new HFA policy framework, targets and schedule Endorsement of regional strategic programme budget for 2000–2001	Publication and marketing of HFA policy framework Seminar for senior public health administrators
5	1998	Implementation of European Alcohol Action Plan (1995–1999) and Action Plan for a Tobacco-free Europe (1997–2001)	Establishment of a European Committee for a Tobacco-free Europe	Implementation

"HEALTH21" Chapter	Action to be taken by:			
	Year	Member States	Regional Committee	Regional Office
7	1999	Translation of HFA policy into local languages	Approval of European Alcohol Action Plan – Second phase (2000–2004) Approval of new HFA indicators	Consultation with various actors and sectors to prepare and distribute issue-specific and/or sector-specific HFA policy documents Seminar for senior public health administrators Meeting of European Health Communication Network and launch of HEALTH21 broadcast series
5				Third European Ministerial Conference on Environment and Health Launch of "Healthy Company" network
4	1999	Participation in poliomyelitis eradication campaign MECACAR Plus (1998–2000)		
7	2000	Marketing of relevant HFA policy principles Monitoring of progress towards HFA Seminars to identify common agendas for intersectoral action for health	Endorsement of regional strategic programme budget for 2002–2003	Consultation on future trends in Europe Forum or major consultation with other sectors as part of series of annual reviews of sector policies Networks of NGOs Seminar for senior public health administrators
6	2000			Conference on a high-priority topic
5	2000	Participation in activities of the European Committee for Health Promotion Development	Endorsement of a "lifestyles action plan"	Development of European Food and Nutrition Security Action Plans
3, 4	2000	Conference on poliomyelitis eradication Conference on a healthy start in life		

Schedule of main events 1998–2005

"HEALTH21" Chapter	Year	Action to be taken by:		
		Member States	Regional Committee	Regional Office
7	2001		Review of results of monitoring progress towards HFA	Seminar for senior public health administrators Joint policy workshops with major organizations
5	2001			Conference on a high-priority topic
7	2002		Endorsement of regional strategic programme budget for 2004–2005	Consultation on future trends Seminar for senior public health administrators
5	2002		Approval of Action Plan for a Tobacco-free Europe – Fourth phase (2003–2007)	
4	2002			Conference on a high-priority topic
7	2003	Evaluation of progress towards HFA		European Advisory Committee on Health Research and Regional Health Development Advisory Council to advise on next update of HFA policy Seminar for senior public health administrators
3	2003			Conference on a high-priority topic
7	2004		Review of results of evaluation of progress towards HFA Endorsement of regional strategic programme budget for 2006–2007	Consultation on future trends Seminar for senior public health administrators
5	2004	Implementation of local environment and health action plans	Approval of European Alcohol Action Plan – Third phase (2005–2009)	Fourth European Ministerial Conference on Environment and Health
7	2005		Approval of renewed regional HFA policy framework	Publication and marketing of HFA policy framework Seminar for senior public health administrators
4	2005			Conference on a high-priority topic

Annex 4

List of abbreviations

AIDS	Acquired immunodeficiency syndrome
BFHI	Baby-Friendly Hospital Initiative
BSE	Bovine spongiform encephalopathy
CAP	Common agricultural policy
CARAK	Central Asian Republics, Azerbaijan and Kazakhstan
CCEE	Countries of central and eastern Europe
CHD	Coronary heart disease
CINDI	Countrywide integrated noncommunicable disease intervention
CIS	Commonwealth of Independent States
CNS	Central nervous system
DALY	Disability-adjusted life year
DFLY	Disability-free life year
DMFT	Decayed, missing or filled teeth
DNA	Deoxyribonucleic acid
DOTS	Directly observed treatment, short course
DTP	Diphtheria/tetanus/pertussis
EBRD	European Bank for Reconstruction and Development
EC	European Commission
ECU	European currency unit
EEA	European Environment Agency
EEHC	European Environment and Health Committee
EME	Established market economy
EU	European Union
EUROHIS	European health interview survey
FAO	Food and Agriculture Organization
FSE	Former socialist economy
GDP	Gross domestic product
GNP	Gross national product
GP	General practitioner
HACCP	Hazard analysis and critical control point
HBV	Hepatitis B virus

HFA	Health for all
HIV	Human immunodeficiency virus
IAEA	International Atomic Energy Agency
IARC	International Agency for Research on Cancer
IDD	Iodine deficiency disease
IFRC	International Federation of Red Cross and Red Crescent Societies
IICC	Interagency Immunization Coordination Committee
MMR	Measles/mumps/rubella
NEHAP	National environment and health action plan
NGO	Nongovernmental organization
NIS	Newly independent state(s)
NMA	National medical association
OECD	Organisation for Economic Co-operation and Development
ORS	Oral rehydration salts
PCF	Polish Consumer Federation
PCTA	Percutaneous transluminal angioplasty
PHC	Primary health care
QALY	Quality-adjusted life year
REMPAN	Radiation Emergency Medical Preparedness and Assistance Network
SCRC	Standing Committee of the Regional Committee
SIDA	Swedish International Development Agency
STD	Sexually transmitted disease
TB	Tuberculosis
UN/ECE	United Nations Economic Commission for Europe
UNAIDS	Joint United Nations Programme on AIDS
UNDP	United Nations Development Programme
UNHCR	Office of the United Nations High Commissioner for Refugees
UNICEF	United Nations Children's Fund
USAID	United States Agency for International Development
WFP	World Food Programme
WHA	World Health Assembly
WHO	World Health Organization
WTO	World Trade Organization

Annex 5

Glossary of terms

Accountability – The result of the process which ensures that decision-makers at all levels actually carry out what they are obliged to do, and that they are made answerable for their actions. The process of setting explicit objectives and targets for health and defining the means of monitoring progress towards them has facilitated the attempt to achieve greater accountability through public disclosure or "transparency". *(2)*

Appropriate health technology – Methods, procedures, techniques and equipment in the field of health that are scientifically valid, adapted to local needs, and acceptable to those who use them and to those for whom they are used, and that can be maintained and utilized with resources the community or the country can afford. *(1)*

Benchmarking – Comparing performance by comparing different aspects of performance with a view to adopting the best methods or performance targets. *(2)*

CINDI – The WHO countrywide integrated noncommunicable diseases intervention programme. Established in 1982, it has the overall aim of improving community health and the quality of life by reducing premature death, disease and disability. The programme is intended to provide CINDI member countries with a framework for the prevention and control of risk factors (e.g. smoking, high blood pressure, abnormal blood lipids and excessive alcohol consumption) which are common to a number of chronic noncommunicable diseases, as well as for addressing the socio-environmental determinants of risk factors. *(2)*

Community action for health – Community action for health refers to collective efforts by communities which are directed towards increasing community control over the determinants of health, and thereby improving health. *(4)*

Community participation – The active involvement of people living together in some form of social organization and cohesion in the planning, operation and control of primary health care, using local, national and other resources. *(1)*

Comprehensive health system – [A health system] that includes all the elements required to meet all the health needs of the population. *(1)*

Control of disease – Reduction of disease incidence, prevalence, morbidity or mortality as a result of deliberate efforts; the disease may no longer be of public health importance, but continued intervention measures are required to maintain the reduction. *(8)*

Determinants of health – The range of personal, social, economic and environmental factors which determine the health status of individuals or populations. The factors which influence health are multiple and interactive. Health promotion is fundamentally concerned with action and advocacy to address the full range of potentially modifiable determinants of health – not only those which are related to the actions of individuals, such as health behaviours and lifestyles, but also factors such as income and social status, education, employment and working conditions, access to appropriate health services, and the physical environments. These, in combination, create different living conditions which impact on health. Achieving change in these lifestyles and living conditions, which determine health status, are considered to be intermediate health outcomes. *(4)*

Disability – In the context of health experience ... any restriction or lack (resulting from an impairment) of ability to perform an activity in the manner or within the range considered normal for a human being. *(1)*

Disease prevention – Measures not only to prevent the occurrence of disease, such as immunization or disease vector control or anti-smoking activities, but also to arrest its progress and reduce its consequences once it is established. *(1)*

Environmental health – Those aspects of human health and disease that are determined by factors in the environment. It also refers to the theory and practice of assessing and controlling factors in the environment that can potentially affect health. Environmental health ... includes both the direct pathological effects of chemicals, radiation and some biological agents, and the effects (often indirect) on health and wellbeing of the broad physical, psychological, social and aesthetic environment, which includes housing, urban development, land use and transport. *(1)*

Equity – Equity in health implies that ideally everyone should have a fair opportunity to attain their full health potential and, more pragmatically, that no one should be disadvantaged from achieving this potential, if it can be avoided. The term *inequity* ... refers to differences in health which are not only unnecessary and avoidable but, in addition, are considered unfair and unjust. *(1)*

Elimination of disease – Reduction to zero of the incidence of a specified disease in a defined geographic area (in "HEALTH 21" this is the European Region of WHO) as a result of deliberate efforts; continued intervention measures are required. *(8)*

Eradication – Permanent reduction to zero of the worldwide incidence of infection caused by a specific agent as a result of deliberate efforts; intervention measures are no longer needed. *(8)*

Gatekeeper function – An accepted role of a particular professional or organizational unit (e.g. at the primary care level) through whom other, often expensive or scarce, care resources are accessed. *(2)*

Gender sensitivity – Incorporation of a gender perspective into health policies and strategies. A gender perspective leads to a better understanding of the facts that influence the health of women and of men. It is not only concerned with biological differences between women and men, or with women's reproductive role, but acknowledges the effects of the socially, culturally and behaviourally determined relationships, roles and responsibilities of men and women, especially on individual, family and community health. *(7)*

Goal – A general aim towards which to strive. Within the health sector WHO has defined the goal of health for all by the year 2000, which means that "as a minimum all people in all countries should have at least such a level of health that they are capable of working productively and participating actively in the social life of the country in which they live". *(3)*

Governance – The system through which society organizes and manages the affairs of diverse sectors and partners in order to achieve its goals. *(7)*

Health – 1. A state of complete physical, mental and social wellbeing and not merely the absence of disease or infirmity. 2. The reduction in mortality, morbidity and disability due to detectable disease or disorder, and an increase in the perceived level of health. The first definition, that of the WHO Constitution, expresses an ideal, which should be the goal of all health development activities (i.e. health as a fundamental human right and a worldwide social goal). It does not, however, lend itself to objective measurement, and for working purposes a narrower definition is required. The second definition is usually used for this purpose (e.g. in health statistics). *(2)*

Health competence – Individual competence to influence factors determining health. *(1)*

Health development – The process of continuous, progressive improvement of the health status of a population. *(3)*

Health education – Consciously constructed opportunities for learning which are designed to facilitate changes in behaviour. *(1)*

Health expectancy – Health expectancy is a population-based measure of the proportion of expected lifespan estimated to be healthful and fulfilling, or free of illness, disease and disability according to social norms and perceptions and professional standards. Examples of health expectancy indicators currently in use are disability-free life years (DFLY) and quality-adjusted life years (QALY). They focus primarily on the extent to which individuals experience a lifespan free of disability, disorders and/or chronic disease. *(4)*

Health for all (HFA) As a minimum, all people in all countries should have at least such a level of health that they are capable of working productively and of participating actively in the social life of the community in which they live (see also Health). *(1)*

Health for all (HFA) policy – An agreed framework for health policy development, based on the values of health for all. *(1)*

Health for all (HFA) target – A European (or national) HFA target is a goal towards which to strive in line with the agreed European (or national) HFA policy. It presupposes a political will to commit a country's resources to the achievement of that goal. *(1)*

Health for all (HFA) value – Health as a human right; equity in health and solidarity; participation and accountability. *(1)*

Health gain – An increase in the measured health of an individual or population, including length and quality of life. *(3)*

Health impact assessment – An estimation of the total, direct and indirect, effects of a policy, programme, service or institution on health status and overall health and socioeconomic development. *(6)*

Health policy – A set of decisions or commitments to pursue courses of action aimed at achieving defined goals and targets for improving health. *(3)*

Health potential – The fullest degree of health that an individual can achieve. Health potential is determined by caring for oneself and others, by being able to make decisions and take control over one's life, and by ensuring that the society in which one lives creates conditions that allow the attainment of health by all its members. *(1)*

Health promotion – The process of enabling individuals and communities to increase control over the determinants of health and thereby improve their health. An evolving concept that encompasses fostering lifestyles and other social, economic, environmental and personal factors conducive to health. *(1)*

Health-promoting hospital – A health-promoting hospital does not only provide high quality comprehensive medical and nursing services, but also develops a corporate identity that embraces the aims of health promotion, develops a health-promoting organizational structure and culture, including active, participatory roles for patients and all members of staff, develops itself into a health-promoting physical environment and actively cooperates with its community. *(4)*

Health-promoting school – A school which aims at achieving healthy lifestyles for the total school population by developing supportive environments conducive to the promotion of health. It offers opportunities for, and requires commitments to, the provision of a safe and health-enhancing social and physical environment. It constantly strengthens its capacity as a healthy setting for living, learning and working. *(2,4)*

Health sector – The health sector consists of organized public and private health services (including health promotion, disease prevention, diagnostic, treatment and care services), the policies and activities of health departments and ministries, health-related nongovernmental organizations and community groups, and professional associations. *(4)*

Health service – Any service which can contribute to improved health or the diagnosis, treatment and rehabilitation of sick people and not necessarily limited to medical or health care services. Also, a formally organized system of established institutions and organizations, the multi-purpose objective of which is to cope with the various health needs and demands of the population. *(3,2)*

Health status – A general term for the state of health of an individual, group or population measured against defined standards. The WHO health indicators provide internationally accepted standards for various aspects of health status. *(3)*

Healthy company – The principles of a healthy company include: a safe working environment; healthy working practices; programmes to promote health and to address psychosocial risk factors at the workplace; health impact assessment for marketed products; and contribution to health and social development in the community.

Health system – A formal structure for a defined population, whose finance, management, scope and content is defined in law and regulations, which provides for services to be delivered to people contributing to their health and health care, delivered in defined settings such as in homes, educational institutions, workplaces, public places, communities, hospitals and clinics and which may affect the physical and psychosocial environment. *(3)*

Healthy city – A city that is continually creating and improving those physical and social environments and expanding those community resources which enable people to mutually support each other in performing all the functions of life and in developing to their full potential. The Healthy Cities project is a long-term development project that seeks to put health on the agenda of decision-makers in the cities of Europe and to build a strong lobby for public health at the local level. The Healthy Cities network is a network of European cities that experiment with new ways of promoting health and improving the environment. *(2)*

Healthy public policy – An explicit concern for health and equity in all areas of policy and an accountability for health impact. The main aim ... is to create a supportive environment to enable people to lead healthy lives. *(1)*

Impairment – In the context of health experience, any loss or abnormality of psychological, physiological, or anatomical structure or function. *(1)*

Indicators – Variables that help to measure [changes in the health situation] directly or indirectly and to assess the extent to which the objectives and targets of a programme are being attained. For the regional HFA targets, both quantitative and qualitative indicators are used. *(1)*

Intergovernmental organization – An organization which is established by intergovernmental agreement. Examples: WHO, Council of Europe, OECD, other specialized agencies of the United Nations system. *(2)*

Intersectoral action – Action in which the health sector and other relevant sectors collaborate for the achievement of a common goal, the contributions of the different sectors being closely coordinated. *(1)*

Investment for health – Investment for health refers to resources which are explicitly dedicated to the production of health and health gain. They may be invested by public and private agencies, as well as by people as individuals and groups. Investment for health strategies are based on knowledge about the determinants of health and seek to gain political commitment to healthy public policies. *(4)*

Lifeskills – Those personal, social, cognitive and physical skills which enable people to control and direct their lives and to develop the capacity to live with and produce change in their environment. *(2)*

Multisectoral action – For practical purposes it is synonymous with intersectoral action, but emphasizing the contribution and accountability of a number of sectors. *(1)*

Nongovernmental organization – A national or internationally based organizational entity such as a citizens' group, an association, a church group or a foundation, that provides an independent and flexible counterbalance to government and the for-profit business sector. *(2)*

Nursing – In its broadest sense, the provision of nursing care to individuals, families or communities in connection with the restoration or preservation of health, and comprising the nursing component of the organized health care and preventive services. Such care may be provided by personnel ranging from the nursing aide to the professional nurse and nurse-midwife. *(9)*

Outcome – In the field of health, the result or impact of policy measures or health interventions in terms of a change in health status or health behaviour. *(2)*

Patients' rights – Patients' basic rights to health in terms of access to care and services, equity in treatment and quality of care. *(2)*

"Polluter pays" principle – The principle incorporated in laws of some countries that those producers who are responsible for pollution should pay the costs of compensation for damage and the cost of "cleaning up" the pollution afterwards. *(3)*

Primary care – The first level of care, generally provided in an ambulatory setting (as opposed to secondary and tertiary care which would normally be hospital-based). *(1)*

Glossary of terms

Primary health care – Primary health care is the central function and main focus of a country's health system, the principal vehicle for the delivery of health care, the most peripheral level in a health system stretching from the periphery to the centre, and an integral part of the social and economic development of a country. *(1)*

Public health – The science and art of preventing disease, prolonging life and promoting mental and physical health and efficiency through organized community efforts. Public health may be considered as the structures and processes by which the health of populations is understood, safeguarded and promoted through the organized efforts of society. *(2,10)*

Public health management –The structures and processes by which the changes necessary for health improvement throughout society are defined and effectively implemented. *(10)*

Public/private mix – The combination of public and private financing and/or delivery of services. *(2)*

Quality of care – The extent to which the care provided, within a given economic framework, achieves the most favourable outcome when balancing risks and benefits. *(1)*

Quality of life – The perception of individuals or groups that their needs are being satisfied and that they are not being denied opportunities to achieve happiness and fulfilment. *(1)*

Regions for Health network – A network of regions in Europe set up by the WHO Regional Office for Europe to achieve change in the thinking about, and action for, the protection, maintenance and promotion of health in regions. It aims to support the commitment of national governments to HFA through the development of appropriate health policies at the regional level. *(2)*

Reorienting health services – Health services reorientation is characterized by a more explicit concern for the achievement of population health outcomes in the ways in which the health system is organized and funded. This must lead to a change of attitude and organization of health services, which focuses on the needs of the individual as a whole person, balanced against the needs of population groups. *(4)*

Reproductive health – Reproductive health addresses the reproductive processes, functions and system at all stages of life. It implies that people are able to have responsible, satisfying and safe sex life and that they have the capability to reproduce and the freedom to decide if, when and how often to do so. Implicit in this last condition is the right of men and women to be informed of and to have access to safe, effective, affordable and acceptable methods of fertility regulation of their choice, and the right of access to appropriate health care services that will enable women to go safely through pregnancy and childbirth and provide couples with the best chance of having a healthy infant. *(5)*

Risk factor – Social, economic or biological status, behaviours or environments which are associated with or cause increased susceptibility to a specific disease, ill health, or injury. *(4)*

Secondary care – Referral services in the first instance provide secondary health care, which is of a more specialized kind than can be offered at the most peripheral level, for example radiographic diagnosis, general surgery, care of women with complications of pregnancy or childbirth, and diagnosis and treatment of uncommon or severe diseases. This kind of care is provided by trained staff in such institutions as district or provincial hospitals. *(1)*

Self-care – All the health care activities carried out by individuals for themselves and their families, including the maintenance of health, prevention of disease, self-diagnosis and self-treatment. *(2)*

Setting for health – The place or social context in which people engage in daily activities in which environmental, organizational and personal factors interact to affect health and wellbeing. *(4)*

Sexual health – The integration of the somatic, emotional, intellectual and social aspects of sexual being, in ways that are positively enriching and that enhance personality, communication, and love. Thus the notion of sexual health implies a positive approach to human sexuality, and the purposes of sexual health care should be the enhancement of life and personal relationships and not merely the counselling and care related to procreation or sexually transmitted diseases. *(5)*

Social capital – Social capital represents the degree of social cohesion which exists in communities. It refers to the processes between people which establish networks, norms and social trust, and facilitate coordination and cooperation for mutual benefit. *(4)*

Social marginalization – The process by which certain vulnerable groups may be prevented from participating fully in social, political and economic life in a community. This occurs when the necessary intersectoral policies and support mechanisms are not in place to enable their full participation. *(1)*

Strategy – A long-term considered and comprehensive course of action that provides the framework for individual activities and events. *(1)*

Supportive environments – Supportive environments for health offer people protection from threats to health, and enable people to expand their capabilities and develop self reliance in health. In a health context ... both the physical and the social aspects of our surroundings. It encompasses where people live, their local community, their home, where they work and play. It also embraces the framework which determines access to resources for living, and opportunities for empowerment. Thus action to create supportive environments has many dimensions: physical, social, spiritual, economic and political. Each of these dimensions is inextricably linked to the others in a dynamic interaction. *(4,1)*

Sustainable development – Development that meets the needs of the present without compromising the ability of future generations to meet their own needs. *(11)*

Tertiary care – Specialized care that requires highly specific facilities and the attention of highly specialized health workers, for example, for neurosurgery or heart surgery. *(1)*

Sources of definitions

(1) *Health for all targets: the health policy for Europe.* Copenhagen, WHO Regional Office for Europe, 1993 (European Health for All Series, No. 4).
(2) *Terminology for the European Health Policy Conference.* Copenhagen, WHO Regional Office for Europe, 1994.
(3) Roberts, J.L. *Terminology for the WHO Conference on European Health Care Reform.* Copenhagen, WHO Regional Office for Europe, 1996.
(4) Nutbeam, D. *Health promotion glossary.* Geneva, World Health Organization, 1998 (document WHO/HPR/HEP/98.1).
(5) *Technical definitions and commentary.* Geneva, World Health Organization, 1994 (briefing document prepared for use at the International Conference on Population and Development, Cairo, Egypt, 5–13 September 1994).
(6) *Planning and managing WHO's programmes.* Geneva, World Health Organization, 1997 (Annex III – Glossary of terms on programme management).
(7) *Health for all in the twenty-first century.* Geneva, World Health Organization, 1998 (document A51/5).
(8) Recommendations of the International Task Force for Disease Eradication. *Morbidity and mortality weekly report (MMWR),* **42**: 1–38 (1993) (Reports and Recommendations RR–16).
(9) *Glossary of health care reform terminology.* Copenhagen, WHO Regional Office for Europe, 1996 (background document compiled for the WHO Consultation of Chief Government Nurses, Reykjavik, 11–13 April 1996).
(10) *Developing public health in the European Region.* Copenhagen, WHO Regional Office for Europe, 1998 (document EUR/RC48/13).
(11) World Commission on Environment and Development. *Our common future.* Oxford University Press, 1987.

Annex 6

Bibliography

Information on further selected reading material may be obtained from the WHO Regional Office. Please send your request to fax: +45 39 17 18 18, marked HEALTH21; or by e-mail to postmaster@who.dk.

Chapter 1

Atlas of mortality in Europe. Subnational patterns 1980/1981 and 1990/1991. Copenhagen, WHO Regional Office for Europe, 1997 (WHO Regional Publications, European Series, No. 75).

Copenhagen Declaration and Programme of Action. World Summit for Social Development 6–12 March 1995. New York, United Nations, 1995.

CORNIA, G.A. *Labour market shocks, psychosocial stress and the transition's mortality crisis, research in progress.* United Nations University/World Institute for Development Economics Research, 1996.

Health for all in the 21st century. Geneva, World Health Organization, 1998 (document WHA 51/5).

Health in Europe 1997. Report on the third evaluation of progress towards health for all in the European Region of WHO (1996–1997). Copenhagen, WHO Regional Office for Europe, 1998 (WHO Regional Publications, European Series, No. 83).

The state of health in the European Community. Luxembourg, Office for Publications of the European Communities, 1996.

The world health report 1998. Life in the 21st century: a vision for all. Geneva, World Health Organization, 1998.

UNITED NATIONS DEVELOPMENT PROGRAMME. *Human development report.* Oxford, Oxford University Press, 1997.

WORLD BANK. *World development report 1997. The state in a changing world.* New York, Oxford University Press, 1997.

World population prospects 1950–2050 (1996 revision). New York, United Nations, 1996.

Chapter 2

DIEREN, W. VAN, ED. *Taking nature into account.* New York, Springer, 1995.

LEVIN, L.S. ET AL. *Economic change, social welfare and health in Europe.* Copenhagen, WHO Regional Office for Europe, 1994 (WHO Regional Publications, European Series, No. 54).

MACKENBACH, J. ET AL. Socioeconomic inequalities in mortality and morbidity in western Europe. *Lancet,* **349:** 1655–1659 (1997).

MARMOT, M.G. Improvement of social environment to improve health. *Lancet,* **351:** 57–60 (1998).

MURRAY, C.J.L. & LOPEZ, A.D. ED. *The global burden of disease.* Boston, MA, Harvard University Press, 1996.

WILKINSON, R. *Unhealthy societies. The afflictions of inequality.* London, Routledge, 1996.

Chapter 3

BARTLEY, M. ET AL. Socioeconomic determinants of health: health and the life course: why safety nets matter. *British medical journal,* **314:** 1194–1196 (1997).

BELLAMY, C., ED. *The state of the world's children 1997.* Oxford, Oxford University Press, 1997.

FERRUCCI, L. ET AL. *Pendulum health and quality of life in older Europeans.* Florence, Istituto Nazionale Ricovero e Cura Anziani, 1995.

Health promotion for old age. London, Eurolink Age, 1998.

Health, economics and development: a people centered approach. Fort Worth, World Federation of Public Health Associations, 1996.

Investing in women's health: central and eastern Europe. Copenhagen, WHO Regional Office for Europe, 1995 (WHO Regional Publications, European Series, No. 55).

KING, A. ET AL. *The health of youth: a cross-national survey.* Copenhagen, WHO Regional Office for Europe, 1996 (WHO Regional Publications, European Series, No. 69).

Labour market changes and job insecurity: a challenge for social welfare and health promotion. Copenhagen, WHO Regional Office for Europe, in press (WHO Regional Publications, European Series, No. 81).

Physical activity and health. A report of the Surgeon General. Washington DC, US Department of Health and Human Services, 1996.

Report of the Fourth World Conference on Women, Beijing, 4–15 September 1995. New York, United Nations, 1995 (document A/CONF.177/20).

Steering Committee on Social Policy – social protection, family policies. Strasbourg, Council of Europe, 1996 (document CDPS CP (96) 3).

Chapter 4

BEECK, E.F. VAN, ET AL. Medical costs and economic production losses due to injuries in the Netherlands. *Journal of trauma*, **42**(6): 1116–1123 (1997).

CHEN, M. ET AL. *Comparing oral health care systems: a second international collaborative study.* Geneva, World Health Organization, 1997 (document WHO/ORH/ICSII/97.1).

LABARTHE, D.R. *Epidemiology and prevention of cardiovascular diseases: a global challenge.* Gaithersburg, Aspen Publishers, 1998.

MANN, J.M. & TARANTOLA, D.J.M. *AIDS in the world (II).* Oxford, Oxford University Press, 1996.

Protocol and guidelines: countrywide integrated noncommunicable diseases intervention (CINDI) programme. Copenhagen, WHO Regional Office For Europe, 1996 (document EUR/ICP/CIND 94 02/PB04).

The Victoria Declaration on Heart Health. Declaration of the Advisory Board – International Heart Health Conference – Victoria, Canada, May 28, 1992. Ottawa, Health and Welfare Canada, 1992.

Treatment of tuberculosis: guidelines for national programmes, 2nd ed. Geneva, World Health Organization, 1997 (document WHO/TB/97.220).

WHO Technical Report Series, No. 862, 1996 (*Hypertension control: report of a WHO Expert Committee*).

Worldwide efforts to improve heart health. A follow-up to the Catalonia Declaration – selected program descriptions. Washington DC, US Department of Health and Human Services, 1997.

Chapter 5

Alcohol – less is better. European Alcohol Action Plan. Copenhagen, WHO Regional Office for Europe, 1996 (WHO Regional Publications, European Series, No.70).

Assessing the health consequences of major chemical incidents – epidemiological approaches. Copenhagen, WHO Regional Office for Europe, 1997 (WHO Regional Publications, European Series, No. 79).

BERTOLLINI, R. ET AL. *Environmental epidemiology. Exposure and disease.* Boca Raton, CRC Press, 1996.

Declaration on Action for Environment and Health in Europe. Second European Conference on Environment and Health, Helsinki, Finland, 20–22 June 1994. Copenhagen, WHO Regional Office for Europe, 1994 (document EUR/ICP/CEH 212).

EDWARDS, G. ET AL. *Alcohol policy and the public good.* Oxford, Oxford Medical Publications, 1994.

EUROPEAN ENVIRONMENT AGENCY. *Europe's environment: the Dobříš assessment*. Luxembourg, Office for Official Publications of the European Communities, 1997.

EUROPEAN ENVIRONMENT AGENCY. *Europe's environment: the second assessment*. Luxembourg, Office for Official Publications of the European Communities, 1998.

EVANS, R.G. ET AL., ED. *Why are some people healthy and others not? The determinants of health of populations*. New York, Aldine De Gruyter, 1994.

Food safety and foodborne diseases. *World health statistics quarterly*, **50**:(1/2):1–154 (1997).

Food safety and globalization of trade in food: a challenge to the public health sector. Geneva, World Health Organization, 1997 (document WHO/FSF/FOS/97.8).

Guidelines for controlling and monitoring the tobacco epidemic. Geneva, World Health Organization, 1998.

HARKIN, A.M. ET AL. *Smoking, drinking and drug-taking in the European Region*. Copenhagen, WHO Regional Office for Europe, 1997.

Health and environment in sustainable development: five years after the Earth Summit. Geneva, World Health Organization, 1997 (document WHO/EHG/97.8).

HOLDER, H.D. & EDWARDS, G. ED. *Alcohol and public policy. Evidence and issues*. Oxford, Oxford Medical Publications, 1995.

LEVIN, L. & ZIGLIO, E. Health promotion as an investment strategy. *Health promotion international,* **11**: 33–40 (1996).

MACARTHUR, I. & BONNEFOY, X. *Environmental health services in Europe 2: Policy options*. Copenhagen, WHO Regional Office for Europe, 1998 (WHO Regional Publications, European Series, No. 77).

PETO, R. ET AL. *Mortality from smoking in developed countries 1950–2000*. Oxford, Oxford Medical Publications, 1994.

Tobacco or health: a global status report. Geneva, World Health Organization, 1997.

WHO EUROPEAN CENTRE FOR ENVIRONMENT AND HEALTH. *Concern for Europe's tomorrow. Health and the environment in the WHO European Region*. Stuttgart, Wissenschaftliche Verlagsgesellschaft, 1995.

Chapter 6

ABLESON, J. & HUTCHISON, B. *Primary health care delivery models: a review of international literature*. Ontario, McMaster University, 1994 (working paper 94-15).

BERGREM, H. ET AL. *1989–1994. Five years with the St Vincent Declaration*. Copenhagen, WHO Regional Office for Europe, 1995.

BOERMA, W.G.W. & FLEMING, D.M. *The role of general practice in primary health care*. London, H.M. Stationery Office, 1998.

Continuous quality development: a proposed national policy. Copenhagen, WHO Regional Office for Europe, 1993 (document EUR/ICP/CLR 059).

Drugs for the elderly, 2nd ed. Copenhagen, WHO Regional Office for Europe, 1997 (WHO Regional Publications, European Series, No. 71).

European health care reforms. The Ljubljana Charter on Reforming Health Care. Copenhagen, WHO Regional Office for Europe, 1996.

Promotion of the rights of patients in Europe. Proceedings of a WHO consultation. The Hague, Kluwer Law International, 1995.

Quality assurance of pharmaceuticals. A compendium of guidelines and related materials. Geneva, World Health Organization, 1997, Vol. 1.

SALTMAN, R.B. & FIGUERAS, J. *European heath care reform. Analysis of current strategies.* Copenhagen, WHO Regional Office for Europe, 1997 (WHO Regional Publications, European Series, No.72).

SALTMAN, R.B. ET AL., ED. *Critical challenges for healthcare reform in Europe*. Buckingham, Open University Press, 1998.

STARFIELD, B. Primary care and health, a cross-national comparison. *Journal of the American Medical Association*, **266**: 2268–2271 (1991).

TARIMO, E. & WEBSTER, E.G. *Primary health care concepts and challenges in a changing world: Alma-Ata revisited.* Geneva, World Health Organization, 1997 (document WHO/ARA/CC/97.1).

WEEL, C. VAN. Primary care: political favourite or scientific discipline? *Lancet*, **348**(11): 1431–1432 (1996).

WHO Technical Report Series, No. 867, 1997 (*The use of essential drugs: model list of essential drugs (ninth list). Seventh report of the WHO Expert Committee*).

WHO Technical Report Series, No. 869, 1997 (*Improving the performance of health centres in district health system: report of a WHO Study Group*).

Chapter 7

BLANE, D. ET AL, ED. *Health and social organization. Towards a health policy for the twenty-first century.* London, Routledge, 1996.

GREEN, G. *Health and governance in European cities. A compendium of trends and responsibilities for public health in 46 Member States of the WHO European Region.* London, European Hospital Management Journal Limited, 1998.

HARRINGTON, P. & RITSATAKIS, A., ED. *European Health Policy Conference: opportunities for the future. Vol. 2. The policy framework to meet the challenges: intersectoral action for health.* Copenhagen, WHO Regional Office for Europe, 1995 (document EUR/ICP/HFAP 94 01/CN01(II)).

Intersectoral action for health. Addressing environment and health concerns in sustainable development. Geneva, World Health Organization, 1997 (document WHO/PPE/PAC/97.1).

KICKBUSCH, I. ET AL., ED. *International handbook on health promotion.* Westport CT, Greenwood Press Inc. (in press).

Our global neighbourhood. Report of the Commission on Global Governance. Oxford, Oxford University Press, 1995.

Renewing the United Nations. A programme for reform. General Assembly, 51st session. New York, United Nations, 1997 (document 97-18979 (E)).

The Jakarta Declaration on leading health promotion into the 21st century. Geneva, World Health Organization, 1997 (document WHO/HPR/HEP/41CHP/BR/97.4).

www.ingramcontent.com/pod-product-compliance
Ingram Content Group UK Ltd.
Pitfield, Milton Keynes, MK11 3LW, UK
UKHW050409240426
12048UKWH00020B/1421